File Copy

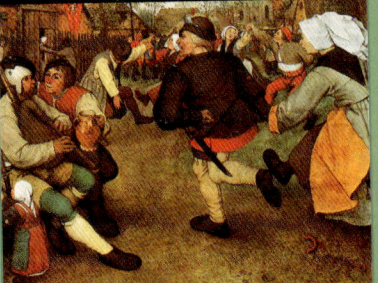

Kenneth Milford

467 Central Park West
New York, NY 10025 212/864-3173
Fax: 212/3167627

P.O. Box 214, 151 E. Housatonic St.
Dalton, MA 01226 413/684-0441

FROM MEDIA TO METAPHOR: ART ABOUT AIDS

Robert Atkins and Thomas W. Sokolowski

Guest Curators

A traveling exhibition organized and circulated by Independent Curators Incorporated, New York

ITINERARY

20 January to 15 March 1992
Emerson Gallery
Hamilton College
Clinton, New York

19 June to 1 August 1992
Center on Contemporary Art
Seattle, Washington

8 September to 6 October 1992
Sharadin Art Gallery
Kutztown University
Kutztown, Pennsylvania

5 November 1992 to 3 January 1993
Musée d'Art Contemporain de Montréal
Montréal, Canada

September to October, 1993
Grey Art Gallery and Study Center
New York University
New York, New York

LENDERS

(Art)^n
Pamela Auchincloss Gallery, New York
Jayne H. Baum Gallery, New York
Ross Bleckner
Kathe Burkhart
Steven Evans
Feature, New York
General Idea
Felix Gonzalez-Torres
Gran Fury
Doug Hammett
The Estate of Keith Haring
Raymond Jacobs
Sidney Janis Gallery, New York
The Estate of Adrian Kellard
Rudy Lemcke
The Robert Mapplethorpe Foundation
Robert Miller Gallery, New York
Donald Moffett
Frank Moore
Ellen B. Neipris
Diane Neumaier
P.P.O.W., New York
Gypsy Ray
Andrea Rosen Gallery, New York
Jane Rosett
John Sapp
Dui Seid
Jo Shane
Rosalind Solomon
Kathy Vargas
Video Data Bank, Chicago
Visual AIDS Artists' Caucus, New York
Andreas Weber
Brian Weil
Zabriskie Gallery, New York

This exhibition, tour, and catalogue are made possible, in part, by a grant from the National Endowment for the Arts and contributions from the ICI Exhibition Patrons Circle.

INDEPENDENT CURATORS INCORPORATED

Board of Trustees

Jan Abrams
Douglas Baxter
Catherine Coleman Brawer
Leslie Cecil
Christo
Anne Ehrenkranz
Arthur Fleischer, Jr.
Tom L. Freudenheim
Gil Friesen
Carol Goldberg
• Agnes Gund
Luisa Kreisberg
Gerrit L. Lansing, Chairman
Suydam R. Lansing
Caral G. Lebworth
Dorothea Rockburne
Robert F. Shapiro
Susan Sollins, Executive Director
Melville Straus
Nina Castelli Sundell
Marcy Syms
Virginia Wright

• Trustee Emerita

Staff

Susan Sollins, Executive Director
Judith Olch Richards, Associate Director
Lyn Freeman, Exhibitions Coordinator
Jack Coyle, Registrar
Anne C. Bornstein, Director of Development
Anne Longnecker, Assistant Exhibitions Coordinator
Alyssa Sachar, Administrative Assistant
Jocelyn H. S. Brayshaw, Development Assistant and Newsletter Coordinator

Interns

Nancy Albin
Anne Le Turnier
Lisa Rapaport

Independent Curators Incorporated, New York, is a non-profit traveling exhibition service specializing in contemporary art. ICI's activities are made possible, in part, by individual contributions and grants from foundations, corporations, and the National Endowment for the Arts.

ACKNOWLEDGMENTS

Many of the artists whose work is included in this exhibition are people with AIDS; some of them are ill and dying. As activists and as artists they bear witness, prodding all of us to address the social and political issues underlying the treatment and care of those who have been diagnosed as HIV-positive and those who have already become gravely ill. AIDS is a difficult subject for Americans to confront; too often the public forum for discussion of AIDS-related issues has been charged with acrimony and prejudice. I trust that this complex exhibition, with its accompanying educational materials, will assist in broadening and deepening public understanding—and that it will lead to the kind of dialogue that is needed to provoke changes in public policy.

I am grateful to ICI's guest curators Robert Atkins and Thomas W. Sokolowski for selecting the exhibition's provocative works—moving and painful, poignant and sad, sometimes beautiful, sometimes difficult to confront.

I am equally grateful to all the artist participants and lenders to the exhibition. I commend ICI's staff—Judith Olch Richards, Jack Coyle, Lyn Freeman, Anne C. Bornstein, Anne Longnecker, Alyssa Sachar, and Jocelyn H. S. Brayshaw. I am also grateful to registrarial assistant Judy Gluck Steinberg, former staff member Mary LaVigne, and interns Minjee Cho and Lisa Rapaport. And, as always, I thank ICI's Board of Trustees for its continuing support.

Susan Sollins
Executive Director

CONTENTS

- 8   The AIDS Crisis: How Can You Help?
- 9   Group Material   AIDS Timeline

- 17   Preface and Dialogue: Robert Atkins and Thomas W. Sokolowski

- 31   (Art)^n
- 32   Ross Bleckner
- 33   Kathe Burkhart
- 34   Nancy Burson
- 35   Steven Evans
- 36   General Idea
- 37   Felix Gonzalez-Torres
- 38   Keith Haring
- 39   Adrian Kellard
- 40   Peter Kunz-Opfersei
- 41   Rudy Lemcke
- 42   Robert Mapplethorpe
- 43   Paul Marcus
- 45   Duane Michals
- 46   Donald Moffett
- 47   Frank Moore
- 40   Ellen B. Neipris
- 49   Diane Neumaier
- 50   Nicholas and Bebe Nixon
- 51   Gypsy Ray
- 52   Rod Rhodes
- 53   Jane Rosett
- 54   John Sapp
- 55   Dui Seid
- 56   Jo Shane
- 57   Rosalind Solomon
- 58   Masami Teraoka
- 59   Max (Torque) = Doug [(Bruno) Hammett]
- 60   Kathy Vargas
- 61   Brian Weil
- 62   David Wojnarowicz
- 63   Thomas Woodruff

- 65   Gran Fury   Video
- 66   Video Data Bank, Chicago
- 67   Visual AIDS Artists' Caucus, New York

- 69   Checklist

THE AIDS CRISIS:
How can you help?

GET THE FACTS
Seek up-to-date information about statistics, trends, scientific and medical advances, government actions and appropriations. Every community has its own AIDS crisis, so keep abreast of local issues. Do research at your library, contact your health department, call the National AIDS Information Clearinghouse (1-800-458-5231).

EDUCATE OTHERS
Listen to people, hear their concerns, provide useful information, urge your employer to conduct seminars and distribute information. Health service organizations can provide trained personnel and audio, video, and printed materials.

SHOW YOU CARE
Join in activities designed to increase awareness, to protest inaction, to pay tribute. Become a buddy, help with food preparation and distribution, volunteer at hospitals and hospices.

CONTRIBUTE
All gifts—even donations of food, clothing, and presents—will help. Honor family and friends on holidays with donations made in their names to AIDS organizations.

SPEAK OUT
Write and call your local and national representatives. Voice your concern for research, health care, educational programs for youth, and risk reduction efforts. Insist on more press coverage. Ask your clergy to speak out publicly about caring.

FIGHT PREJUDICE
Open discussions about AIDS and insist that all people with AIDS merit help.

PROTECT YOURSELF AND RESPECT OTHERS
Talk with sexual partners about AIDS and never initiate sexual activity while "under the influence." Use condoms and spermicidal lubricants. Never share needles or other drug paraphernalia.

REMEMBER
All people living with AIDS are innocent. Let love and caring overcome fear. Commit yourself to providing for all people equally. Envision a cure and work for it.

Produced for *Day Without Art 1991* by
Visual AIDS Artists' Caucus
131 West 24th Street #3
New York, NY 10011
Tel 212-206-6758
Fax 212-206-8159

quest for $833,800 made
Dr. Jim Curran from the NIH
ual budget to study the new
y cancer" is denied.

This years's Reagan Budget calls for
the slashing of at least 1,000 grants from
the National Institute of Health (NIH),
the federal agency that controls research
and prevention of this new epidemic.

The Gay Men's Health Crisis
(GMHC) is founded in New York
City. GMHC is a grass roots
organization of volunteers which
seeks to provide information
and support services through
its buddy program, education,
counseling, legal services and
advocacy for people with AIDS.

"Homosexual Plague Srikes New Victims"
is the title of an article in the August 19th
Newsweek magazine. The piece is inspired
by news from the National Cancer Institute
describing growing evidence that hemophiliacs are showing AIDS-related symptoms.
The article reports, "the homosexual plague
has started spilling over into the general
population."

In October, the Centers for Disease Control
(CDC), in Atlanta, initiates the reporting of KS
(Kaposi's sarcoma) and PCP (Pneumocystis
carinii pneumonia) nationwide.

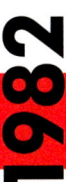

1982

The first Wall Street Journal
article on AIDS is printed only
after 23 heterosexual men and
women are diagnosed with
the disease.

S, as an acronym for Acquired Immune Deficiency Syndrome,
aces earlier namings of the syndrome: GRID (Gay Related Immune
ciency); CAID (Community Acquired Immune Deficiency);
(Acquired Immune Deficiency).

San Franciscans hold a candlelight march,
one of the earliest mass demonstrations of
outrage at the lack of response by medical
and governmental agencies to the progres-
sion of AIDS.

Art Direction: James Morrow

Reprinted from *Shift*, December 1990.

This fragment of **Group Material's** *AIDS TIMELINE is presented as a collaborative project for* DAY WITHOUT ART 1990 *by* **Visual AIDS** *and the following publications in their December issues:* **Afterimage, Art & Auction, Art in America, Art New England, Artforum, Arts, Contemporanea, High Performance, October, Parkett,** *and* **Shift**.

The Names Project is founded by Cleve Jones in San Francisco. The Names Project AIDS Memorial Quilt is displayed at the 1987 Gay and Lesbian March on Washington.

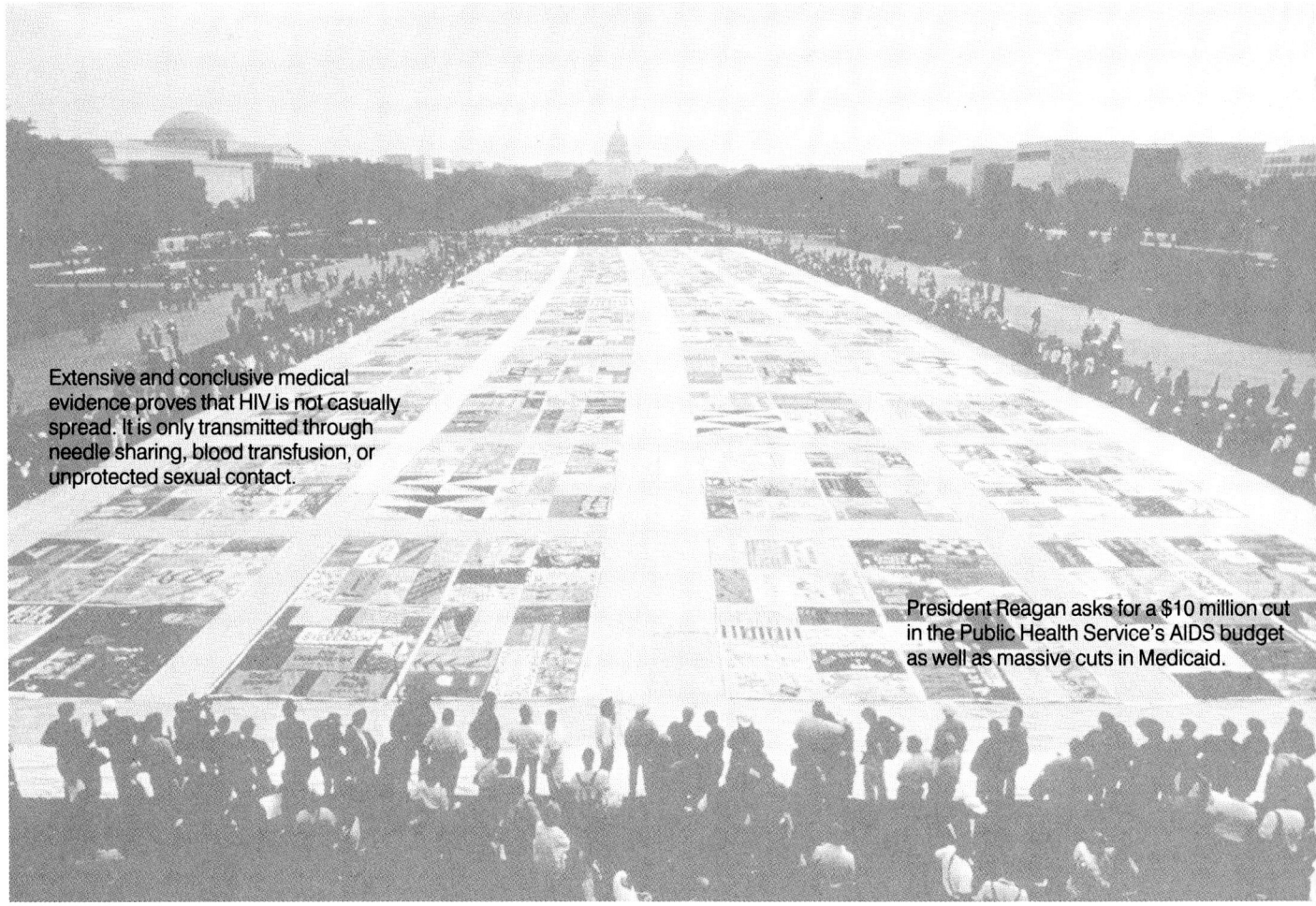

Extensive and conclusive medical evidence proves that HIV is not casually spread. It is only transmitted through needle sharing, blood transfusion, or unprotected sexual contact.

President Reagan asks for a $10 million cut in the Public Health Service's AIDS budget as well as massive cuts in Medicaid.

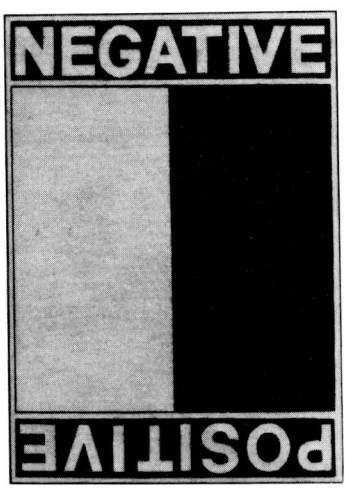 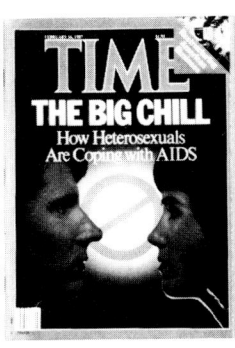 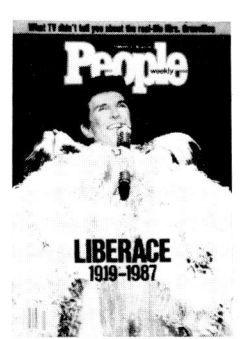 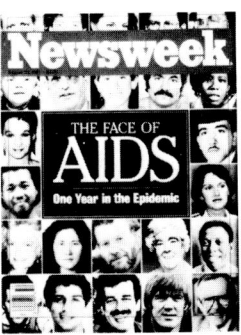

1987

The President orders mandatory AIDS testing for all immigrants and federal prisoners. His Education Secretary, William Bennet, presses for even more extensive mandatory testing while Surgeon General C. Everett Koop joins most public health authorities in opposing this as a wasteful process.

The federal government finally begins to deal with treatment and drug trials. But AIDS drug trials, like many others, exclude women, people of color, poor people, people in rural areas, I.V. drug users, hemophiliacs, prisoners, and children, many of whom die from preventable and treatable illness.

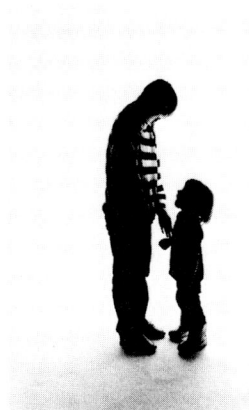

The proportion of women with AIDS increases between 1982 and 1986 from 12% to 26%. Even this statistic is low because most women with AIDS die undiagnosed, with infections specific to women such as severe vaginitis, pelvic inflammatory disease, or cervical cancer, all unrecognized as AIDS related by the Centers for Disease Control.

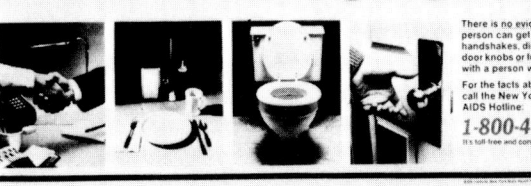

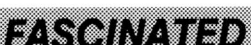

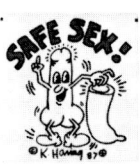

Condom manufacturers produce their first television commercials and all three major national networks refuse to broadcast them.

The Names Project, photo by Tom Alleman · "Black / White", Brad Melamed · "Anonymous and 5 Year Old Son", Ann Meredith · New York City Health Department subway poster · "Selections From The Disco, Various BPM, 1979-1990", Steven Evans · condom case: Keith Haring · art direction: James Morrow

Reprinted from *October*, December 1990.

This fragment of Group Material's AIDS TIMELINE is presented as a collaborative project for DAY WITHOUT ART 1990 by Visual AIDS and the following publications in their December issues: Afterimage, Art & Auction, Art in America, Art New England, Artforum, Arts, Contemporanea, High Performance, October, Parkett, and Shift.

After 444 days in captivity, 51 members of the American Foreign Service who have been held as hostages by Iranian students in Tehran are released.

President Ronald Reagan proposes to slash federal education, welfare, housing, and health budgets. In his budget the National Institutes of Health, the federal agency responsible for testing drugs and treatments, is cut by $127 million.

Kaposi's sarcoma, (KS), an extremely rare form of cancer has been diagnosed in 26 homosexual men. Medical officals are mystified by the occurrence of this disease in men under the age of 50 – a group virtually unknown to have been affected by this disease.

The media portrays the early patients with "gay cancer" as promiscuous homosexual males. The syndrome is partly blamed on "lifestyle" or sexual preference. The risk of sexually transmitted diseases and the transmission of a "new" agent were linked at this early stage.

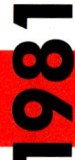

1981

The Sentinel, a San Francisco gay-community newspaper, publishes a small article on June 26, entitled "Unique Pneumonia Strikes Gay Men." The article reports, "Health officials said recently that there has been a mysterious outbreak of pneumonia among gay males."

"Poppers," or amyl nitrates, are considered a possible cause of "gay cancer" in the investigation of the new syndrome in an effort to prove the "lifestyle" theory.

An article by Bobbi Campbell R.N., is published in the San Francisco Sentinel. This is the first public testimonial by a person with Kaposi's sarcoma. That same issue compares governmental and medical response to AIDS with these agencies' earlier responses to the outbreak of Legionnaires disease. In 1976, the federal government instituted emergency measures to find the cause of Legionnaires which had affected 29 people in Philadelphia. Comparatively, there has been no federal response to on-going early "gay cancer" cases.

•med drug company
•midine to prevent AIDS-
•f I.V. Pentamidine by 300%.
$6.00 to $1.80 per dose.

•d and Drug
•g approval
•accelerates

•ching bands

•esident Bush
•October 1987,
•he content of
•a plan that

Arcadia, Florida, bans two young
•ol. Only after a victorious federal
•onths later, their family home is
The family is forced to relocate

Only 89 patients have recieved Trimetrexate, a costly drug believed to be more potent against PCP than Bactrim or I.V. Pentamidine. Since AIDS drug trials, like many others, exclude women, people of color, poor people, people in rural areas, I.V. drug users, hemophiliacs, prisoners, and children, many of these people still die from preventable and treatable illnesses.

The Museum of Modern Art in New York City exhibits Nicholas Nixon's portraits of People With AIDS. Nixon's series of photographs chronicles his subjects as their illness progresses. ACT UP/NY states:

"...in portraying PWAs as people to be pitied or feared, as people alone and lonely, we believe that this work perpetuates general misconceptions about AIDS without addressing the realities of those of us living everyday with this crisis as PWAs or as people who love PWAs.

...We believe that the representation of People With AIDS affects not only how the viewers will perceive PWAs outside the museum, but, ultimately, crucial issues of AIDS funding, legislation, and education."

photo: Rolf Sjogren   design: James Morrow

Reprinted from *Afterimage*, December 1990.

This fragment of Group Material's AIDS TIMELINE is presented as a collaborative project for DAY WITHOUT ART 1990 by Visual AIDS and the following publications in their December issues: Afterimage, Art & Auction, Art in America, Art New England, Artforum, Arts, Contemporanea, High Performance, October, Parkett, and Shift.

As the market for AIDS drugs increases, Lyph competes for federal approval of aerosol Pent related pneumonia (PCP), and raises the cost The cost to actually make the drug drops from

Two thousand AIDS activists "seize control" of the U.S. Fo Administration to protest the laggardly pace of the AIDS dr process. As a result of this demonstration the government the approval process by an average of three years.

$193 million is allocated for military ma in this year's federal budget.

Senator Dan Quayle of Indiana is selected by Vice P as his running mate on the Republican ticket. Since Quayle has voted five times in Congress to restrict educational material on AIDS. He has also opposed would supply AZT to impoverished people with AID

Yolanda Serrano, Executive Director of the Association for Drug Abuse Prevention and Treatment, announces that ADAPT will distribute clean needles to prevent the spread of HIV among I.V. drug users in New York City. In response to this act of "civil disobedience," the New York City Department of Health freezes ADAPT's money and shuts down their office for 48 hours. A month later, Governor Mario Cuomo revises his stand and supports experimental needle exchange.

Congressman William Dannemeyer endorses California State Proposition 102 which would make anonymous testing illegal and force tho who test HIV positive to disclose the names of their sexual partners. It is voted on and defeat by a margin of more than two to one.

The DeSoto County School District brothers with AIDS from attending s court suit are they re-admitted. Two burned down by unidentified arson to another city.

1988

PREFACE

From Media to Metaphor is an exhibition of artists' responses to the AIDS crisis. Because no single artistic voice or viewpoint is capable of grappling with the complexity of the epidemic, we have selected works by dozens of artists that, en masse, evoke the impact of AIDS on American society and psyches.

It is clear that one cannot talk about AIDS—or art about AIDS—without raising contentious issues of sex and sexual identity, public health and private morality. In order to discuss these matters, the following essay assumes the unconventional form of a dialogue focused on AIDS and art's place in the midst of the crisis. Commentary about the works in the show, grounded in both social conditions and aesthetic concerns, can be found in another part of this catalogue. We believe that our dialogue is more likely to raise difficult questions than to provide easy answers.

In the face of a deepening and ongoing catastrophe, there is little room for the sonorous voice of authority, including the art historian's often reflexive impulse to categorize. The ebb and flow of our dialogue is intended as an analogue of AIDS-related social conditions that are continually—and messily—in flux. We hope that in conjunction with the exhibited art it will provide information, stimulate action to stem the spread of HIV infection, and foster more humane treatment for people living with AIDS.

—Robert Atkins and Thomas W. Sokolowski

ART ABOUT AIDS: TWO VOICES—MULTIPLE CONTEXTS

Thomas Sokolowski: In the fall of 1987 when I was working on *Morality Tales: History Painting in the 1980s*, an ICI exhibition of large-scale paintings about contemporary social issues, there were very few artists making art about AIDS.

Robert Atkins: Now there are so many—perhaps 500 professional artists in the United States who put AIDS at the center of their work.

While organizing the exhibition we certainly had the sense that one artist's work might stand for many who are dealing with similar aspects of the crisis.

When we began thinking about this show in early 1989, we also believed that not only was too little work about AIDS being shown, but that artists were sometimes penalized for making it.

Meaning much of it wasn't—and isn't—saleable. What strikes me about the many projects produced for the 1989 Day Without Art [the national day of action and mourning in response to the AIDS crisis] is that so many were temporary, site-specific pieces. Some of the first AIDS-related works, then, were specifically commissioned installations that no longer exist.

And the corollary is that painters—operating in the most conservative, most commodified of art-making media—began to make work about AIDS after the installation artists you've referred to, and three to four years after the first photographers. The first major bodies of AIDS-inspired works were produced by photographers working in the modern,

documentary tradition. They tried to combat the horrific representations of people with AIDS (PWAs) made by photo-journalists and the electronic media.

That's where the *media* of the show's title comes from; it doesn't mean art-making mediums like paint-on-canvas or cast bronze.

AIDS was named in 1982; the first wave of photographers wasn't active until at least 1985 and not exhibited until 1988. The entire field of depicting AIDS had been left to the largely unsympathetic mainstream media. Perhaps the major exception was the NAMES Project Quilt, which debuted in 1987. Its heartbreaking—and unthreatening—emphasis on memorialization helped make the subject of AIDS palatable to those who read about it in *People* magazine. In retrospect, it's not surprising that so many photographers felt the urge early on to create sympathetic—or positive—images of PWAs, in conscious opposition to the exploitive and grisly media images that depicted them as if they were starving Ethiopian babies. Until the *Rosalind Solomon: Portraits in the Time of AIDS* exhibition at the Grey Art Gallery and the AIDS component of Nicholas Nixon's retrospective, *Portraits of People*, at the Museum of Modern Art in 1988, this photo-work was still rather underground.

One of the chief responses to those shows was acrimony. Whether perceived as negative or positive, these pictures occasioned an outcry among some activists. The objectors saw—and still see—Nixon's serial portraits as lacking in social context and creating emaciated monsters out of PWAs. But such exhibitions were rare in 1988 and these photos allowed the faces of individual PWAs to be seen. PWAs were regarded as individuals, rather than as statistics.

At least these photographers documented the reality of who PWAs are. Of the few TV movies about AIDS, for instance, only *An Early Frost* (1985) and *Our Sons* (1991) featured gay PWAs—and none have focused on drug users or their sex partners. Instead we see heroic depictions of 'innocent' victims who contracted the HIV virus through blood transfusions. The divisive media constructions of

'guilty' and 'innocent' victims were precisely what these initial, well-intentioned photographers were confronting.

Solomon's photographs were also more palatable than Nixon's because, in many cases, the PWAs she photographed look healthy—as so many HIV+ people or PWAs do. Nixon's work was more abrasive. For the first time, in a mainstream art context, viewers saw images of people who were visibly ill. Many people didn't want to see them and accused Nixon of undermining PWAs whose lives are difficult enough.

When a group from ACT UP [the AIDS Coalition to Unleash Power] leafletted Nixon's Museum of Modern Art show, their broadside called in part for images of PWAs "who are loving, vibrant, sexy, and acting up." Yet some PWAs find Nixon's work a powerfully realistic representation of themselves. Solomon's and Nixon's works also suffer from the inherent limitations of the modern, documentary, black-and-white tradition that includes both photojournalism and so-called art photography. As a medical, political, and ethical phenomenon, AIDS is staggeringly complex. In an uncaptioned photograph, it's sometimes impossible to determine what's going on. Is it about AIDS? Or is this simply a generic picture of a young woman in a hospital? The context in which you see the work—an exhibition, a magazine, or a political demonstration—may largely determine its meaning.

The imaging of AIDS by artists almost immediately brought the conflicting needs of different audiences out in the open. On one hand, there was an ill-informed 'general' public and, on the other, insiders including PWAs and activists. How could there be one kind of image that would serve everyone's needs?

There is more agreement on another matter of representation, of 'positive' imagery—that is, the depiction of PWAs in language, and their preference for being called "people with AIDS" rather than "AIDS victims." Max Navarre, who was one of the founders of the PWA Coalition, said "I'm a person with a condition, I'm not that condition." Until the PWA movement emerged out of the Denver conference in 1983, there were no organized outlets for the views of those living with the syndrome.

Photographer Gypsy Ray would later respond to this void by insetting the comments of PWAs into the mats surrounding her pictures. Nicholas and Bebe Nixon's new book, *People with AIDS* (1991), includes extensive interviews. Both Ray and Nixon interviewed the care-givers and loved ones of PWAs, as well as PWAs themselves.

There's the cliché that in ten years everybody will be committed to doing something about AIDS because we will all know somebody who is HIV-infected. The present lack of connection between the public at large and PWAs, as expressed through language, is also something the Canadian art collective General Idea has been exploring in their artworks based on Robert Indiana's famous *Love* icon. Since 1987, they've appropriated Indiana's format and converted the four letters of "love" into the four letters of "AIDS." Some regarded it as a cheap trick—love being the emblematic word and activity of the '60s, and AIDS its corollary in the '80s. In fact, their stated intention was to "domesticate" the word, to communicate that AIDS is an unfortunate part of everyday life and not merely scientific jargon.

One purpose of this show is to present audiences with information about AIDS, as well as contemporary art.

Information about AIDS prevention, treatment, and community resources for PWAs will be available so that if a well-informed visitor comes to the show, he or she will find new information. And if you are someone who has never seen a PWA or considered the dilemmas that face PWAs, then this exhibition will provide information about that, too.

The show suggests a number of possible human and artistic responses to the epidemic. A problem with some AIDS exhibitions is that they have not overtly promoted activism—whether that means urging the public to contribute money or time for the care of PWAs, or to write letters to Congress, or to demonstrate at the Centers for Disease Control. Because all sorts of people in urban centers are affected by AIDS—people of color, gay and lesbian people, the health-care community, to name a few—the appeal of a show like this might extend beyond the usual audience for

contemporary art. We want to make sure that informational and educational resources are available.

And that the exhibition speaks as directly as possible.

We've deliberately chosen works that are not 'coded' in the sometimes difficult-to-decipher, visual language of historical or contemporary art. We hope that these works will speak to varied audiences.

By its nature, this show engages contemporary art that is inextricably and immediately linked to its social context. Much of the art derives from artists' hands-on experience with PWAs—such as Paul Marcus's lengthy involvement with a young mother in the Bronx who subsequently died, or Dui Seid's experience as a home-care attendant for PWAs.

Many of the pieces in the show have also generated debate, beyond the narrow confines of the art world, about the representation of AIDS. Nancy Burson's poster, *Visualize This.*, for instance, is an object of visualization for PWAs. She took photo-microscopic images of an HIV-infected and a healthy T-cell and made a poster from them. Its meaning was debated by funders from whom she sought production costs, and by people who saw the work wheat-pasted on New York walls. Detractors felt that it placed the responsibiility for the AIDS crisis on PWAs rather than on the government. This position may be a polarizing example of either/or thinking not necessarily in the best interests of PWAs. Some PWAs employ Eastern and Western medicine, visualize and meditate, and participate in demonstrations as well.

Many of the artists in the show are PWAs; too many others have died of HIV-related causes. Their AIDS experiences, given form in art, teach by example. Being an artist allows you to take your life experiences—positive or negative—and make them the basis of your work. The shock of discovering your HIV+ status—or that of someone close—might be transformed into art.

Or perhaps action.

Wherever the show travels, its hosts will produce a local component that can be used as an organizing tool. The local component also allows for a kind of update, an opportunity to create dialogue between artists, care-givers, and service organizations.

It can give artists the opportunity not just to exhibit their work about AIDS, but to investigate local AIDS conditions. Every community has its own epidemic.

As we conduct this discussion in mid-May 1991, the Whitney Biennial has just concluded. Critics have noted that its thematic undercurrent is the AIDS crisis. The works range from the very pointed *AIDS Timeline* by Group Material [fragments are reproduced in this catalogue], to more subjective and indirect allusions that can be read as a generalized sense of angst, sadness, or anger.

A sort of emotional barometer.

This emotional barometer might be social, as well as psychological. The members of General Idea are Canadian, and they split their time between New York and Toronto. They see their work as very different from American art about AIDS. They feel that they can make art about what Elizabeth Kubler-Ross, in her book *On Death and Dying*, described as the third stage (acceptance) of coming to terms with death, partly because the Canadian government has been so much more responsive to the needs of PWAs.

AIDS is an emotional barrage. In the face of so much death comes overwhelming grief and anger. Thomas Woodruff spent months painting self-portraits of himself as a crying clown. The texts of David Wojnarowicz's works are shockingly direct in their rage. The emotional range of recent AIDS art seems to be widening. The anger of a work by Donald Moffett that reads "Call the White House and tell Bush we're not all dead yet" is tempered by a defiant and liberating irony. What some viewers might dismiss as mere propaganda is leavened by mordant wit.

Moffett's subversive use of media and advertising techniques is also very contemporary. How does art about AIDS relate to art about earlier social crises?

The art world has changed drastically during the past two decades. Thanks in large part to feminist-inspired pressures of the '70s, even very mainstream artists acquired 'permission' to abandon abstraction, to make figurative art, and still remain in the mainstream. To cite just one example, Leon Golub made compelling paintings twenty-five years ago about soldiers in Vietnam, and later about mercenaries in Central America. One of the reasons that the earlier work didn't get much attention was its distance from the stylistic mainstream. Now there is no single ruling mode of art-making. The socially engaged coexists with the most determinedly formalist art; abstract painting shares the spotlight with artworks on billboards. The current pluralism makes it possible to hear from those who have never before been allowed to speak. These marginalized voices are highly attuned to the tremendous social problems facing the United States. In many cases, the artists have experienced those problems, including AIDS.

Art that responds to social crisis brings to mind art produced in Siena during the Black Death of the fourteenth century. It tended to be emblematic and to adhere to a very specific canon of beliefs promulgated by the Roman Catholic Church. Prayers to Christ himself, or to the Blessed Virgin or saints who would act as intercessors to God on one's behalf, would be accompanied by vows. If a town was spared from the plague, an illness cured, a child born healthy, prayers of thanksgiving would be linked to the production of an ex voto painting as a sign of gratitude. Thus the artwork was made afterward; it was retrospective.

And it also embodied the collective beliefs of those in power, in this case representatives of the Church and State. It seems safe to say that an artist is always commissioned to represent a patron's point of view.

Closer in time were the FSA [Farm Securities Administration] photographs commissioned by the federal government to document the rural woes of the Depression. They were intended to prove whether the troubles that government officials in Washington, D.C. had heard about were as bad as reports indicated.

There's something like that happening now on a modest scale. The Library of Congress is collecting documentary photographs about AIDS.

During the Depression, the government's role was not so adversarial. The impact of the economic crisis was being documented by photographers and ameliorated by New Deal legislation.

The overt depoliticization of postwar American art—which can in part be traced to artists' and intellectuals' revulsion to the cynical Hitler-Stalin pact of 1939—dominated American art of the 1940s, '50s, and '60s. Postwar existentialism was translated into the psychologically-oriented abstract art of the mainstream. Today it's difficult to imagine abstraction's stronghold on art production. During that period, overt political expression—such as Warhol's anti-Nixon prints for the McGovern campaign—rarely surfaced in the work of well-known artists.

Warhol is certainly the progenitor of so much media-inspired, activist art about AIDS, whether it's intended for the gallery or the street. He understood that the modus operandi of Madison Avenue might be applicable to SoHo. Gran Fury—whose very name evokes a '60s-model Plymouth—makes their art and politics inseparable, including their manipulation of the media as a sort of stand-in for audiences who can read about, rather than see, the work. One buzzword of the '80s was strategy, and sometimes the strategy became the artwork's concept.

And there are other kinds of strategizing as well.

The art world has rarely displayed such solidarity as it has in connection with AIDS. The commitment has come from artists, critics, and curators. Art is also a useful fund-raising tool. Art Against AIDS auctions donated artworks to raise money for AmFar [American Foundation for Aids Research] for medical research. At Visual AIDS in New York, art is used as an educational tool. Another Visual AIDS group in San Francisco raises money to help PWA-artists buy art supplies. There are collectives like Art+, in New York, which produce programs, as well as demonstrate. This list only scratches the surface.

Some of the art world's solidarity about AIDS also derives from the many attempts to censor art about AIDS, particularly explicitly sexual imagery produced by gay men. Openly gay and lesbian artists are commonplace in the mainstream art world. If the AIDS epidemic had initially hit IV-drug users, it would have been difficult to predict art-world involvement. This is largely a matter of class; professional artists tend to be middle-class. An unfortunate by-product of gay and lesbian leadership of AIDS awareness and activism efforts is that it plays into the hands of those who cynically manipulate homophobia—sometimes by attempting to censor publicly funded art. Art about AIDS frequently invokes political outrage or attitudes toward sexual activity and that's led to some bruising controversies. The first involved an attempted withdrawal of NEA support for *Witnesses: Against Our Vanishing*, the AIDS exhibition that was John Frohnmayer's first crisis after he became chairman of the National Endowment for the Arts in late 1989. AIDS was also the subtext of the Robert Mapplethorpe controversy and trial, although homosexuality was the censors' pretext.

An early and articulate voice in writing about AIDS and sexual repression was Simon Watney, the author of *Policing Desire: Pornography, AIDS, and the Media* (1987). Although the book focused on Britain, the handwriting on the wall is disturbingly clear. A government-condoned sexual panic exacerbated by AIDS has created a climate in which the British government is attempting to recriminalize the activities of sexual minorities.

What's most surprising is that the virulent assault on American freedom of expression has been so effective. It's partly a problem of misleading sound bites and misrepresentations akin to the characterization of a publicly sited AIDS artwork by Gran Fury called *Kissing Doesn't Kill: Greed and Indifference Do* as an "enticement to homosexuality." And painter Kathe Burkhart has depicted Elizabeth Taylor, AIDS fund-raiser and activist extraordinaire, defending herself against "charges" of having AIDS—as if having AIDS were a crime and would render her generosity suspect.

The Right understands the power of symbols. Because symbols are richly ambiguous, they are easily manipulated. Look at the Cross: it can stand for the most liberal theology of the Unitarian Church and its virtual opposite, the Ku Klux Klan. Art itself—as opposed to individual artworks—is also symbolic. It partakes of the authority of the gallery or the museum—from a work's literal and figurative location on a pedestal or in a frame. For many people, art is a potent enigma and if it's perceived as an attack on long-held values or beliefs, then it's understandably frightening.

If some want to prescribe what kind of art artists should make, others are likely to prescribe what kind of art this show should present.

It is likely to incite criticism from several directions. For some viewers the imagery may be overly explicit. Others would curate a show like ours with exclusively didactic intentions, an explicit agenda that every artwork about AIDS must overtly concern itself with ending the crisis. This seems too doctrinaire.

How can anyone anticipate the effect an artwork—or a group of artworks—will have on a variety of audiences?

Maybe this exhibition is unusual because we acknowledge a sometimes blurry divide between art and activism; we don't always see them as synonymous. Good politics do not necessarily make for good art.

Bad political art is bad politics *and* bad art.

There are certain subjects that a society may deem unrepresentable. That is, they cannot—or should not—be addressed by artists because they are regarded, in some sense, as sacred.

As a [Jewish] child, it was clear to me that the Holocaust was something that couldn't—or shouldn't—be represented. Its awesome hideousness rendered it unimaginable. But that prohibition seemed to disappear over time, and there was a point in the '50s or '60s when plans for Holocaust memorials began to be formulated. Originally they were to be dematerialized and abstract, in the form of an eternal

flame, for instance. But by the '70s, George Segal could make his figurative sculpture-memorial. Time must have lessened the shock and undermined the taboo against representation.

Memorials have assumed so many forms. Rudy Lemcke's proposal for an AIDS memorial in San Francisco is abstract—a meditative Zen garden. The Vietnam Memorial is simply a black wall with names on it. It's not inherently horrific, but that palpable roll-call of 56,000 names is extremely moving. How can we not be touched when we see all those names, even if we don't read them, even if we don't know anybody who died? Art allows public and private grief to coexist. When you rub your finger over your brother's name it becomes a personal act of mourning. But it is also about a nation's loss—its loss of naivete, of the glorious promise of post-World War II America.

The names inscribed on the Vietnam Memorial make it shockingly specific but as ordinary looking as a telephone book. I saw the memorial for the first time in 1987, the day before the NAMES Project Quilt appeared on the Washington Mall. A brilliant work of community art, the Names Project Quilt vividly testifies to individual diversity. In an entirely different way, one is also aware that each of the 56,000 names on the Vietnam Memorial stands for the passing of an individual.

An extraordinary thing about the quilt is the collective quality of the viewing experience as it travels from place to place. Of course, it is profoundly touching to see someone kneeling and crying at a lover's—or child's—quilt-square. But then your own tears might flow, quite independent of the specific thing being seen.

Again, the personal and the collective.

There are two sentences that Susan Sontag wrote in the first pre-AIDS version of *Illness as Metaphor* (1977) that suggest a split that cannot be bridged. She wrote, "Everyone who is born holds dual citizenship, in the kingdom of the well and in the kingdom of the sick. Although we all prefer to use only the good passport, sooner or later each of us is obliged, at least for a spell, to identify ourselves as citizens of that other place." When one is in one kingdom, one cannot even contemplate the other. And yet, at some point, our position will shift. The same thing is true of art, in the sense that art too can be so rarefied, so removed from so many people's daily lives. If you're uninterested in art, you may not understand—or care to understand—what artists are doing, and what it might mean.

You're speaking in metaphors. Can art save lives?

Not directly. But it can help the rest of us live.

—September 1991

(ART)ⁿ

Messiah, 1987
PHSCologram sculpture
6 panels
96 × 60 × 14 inches overall

"We knew we wanted to used colorized CAT scans of an anonymous AIDS patient.... When we received the CAT scans, we discovered that the patient was named Messiah. At that moment we knew that the sculpture had to be in the shape of a crucifix. We decided to focus on hope, chance, and death as the sub-themes of the work. The face of death [is] cast in glass, the hand of hope [is] a piece of folk art found in Wisconsin, the dice [are] animated, and the AIDS virus [is]...a 'virtual' sculpture, existing only as PHSCologram [the group's patented, three-dimensional imaging system]."

(Art)ⁿ is a Chicago-based collaborative group dedicated to exploring the interface of art and science. Group members are Randy Johnson, Stephan Meyers, Dan Sandin, Ellen Sandor, and Jim Zanzi.

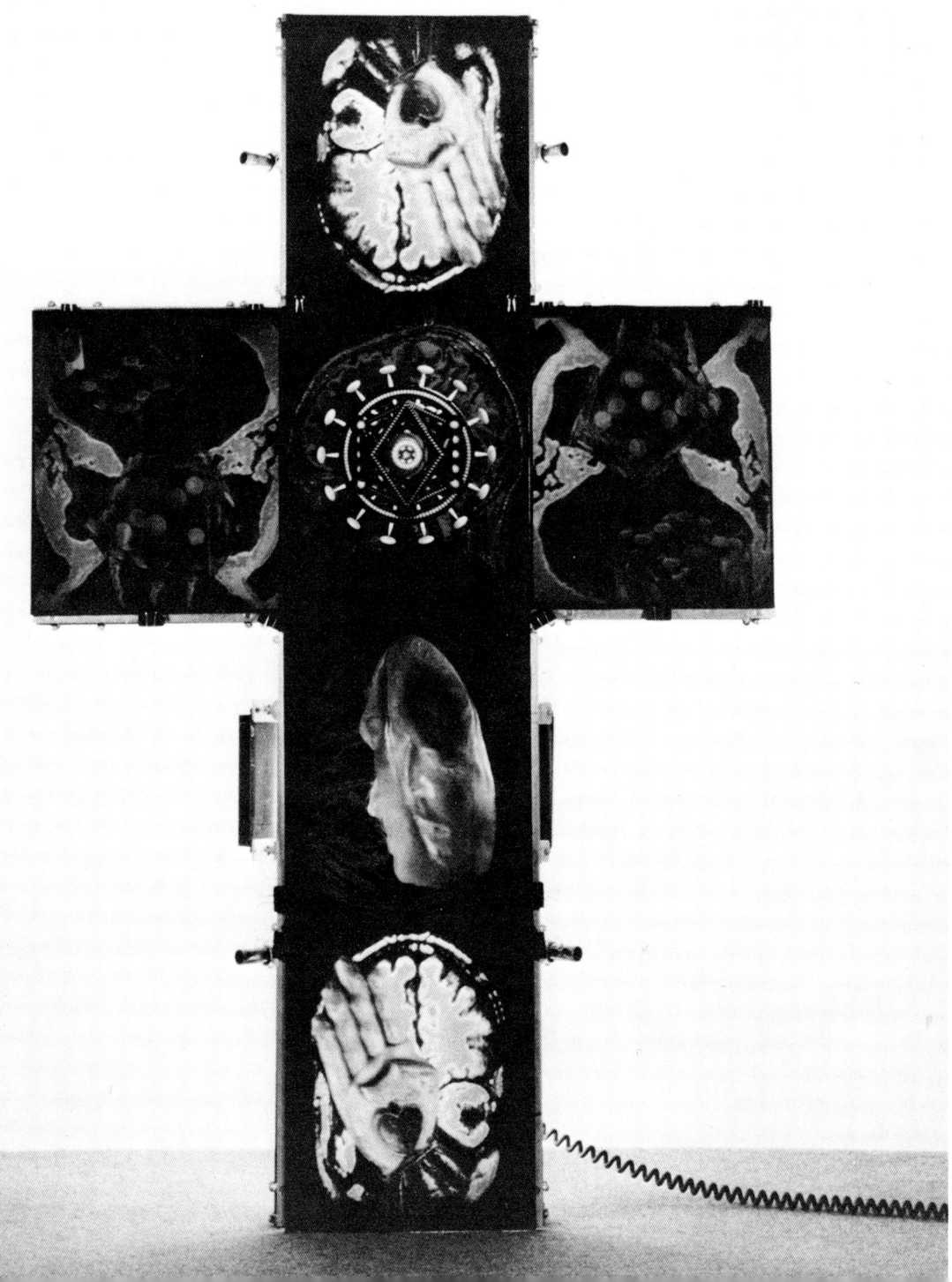

ROSS BLECKNER

Study for Internal Medicine, 1991
Oil on linen
4 panels, 18 × 14 inches each
36 × 28 inches overall

Ross Bleckner's melancholic images of dimmed lights, funerary urns, and numerical renderings of the total of HIV-related fatalities in the United States were first shown in 1985. They were among the first paintings about AIDS to be exhibited. Bleckner's recent work alludes to microscopic images of cells.

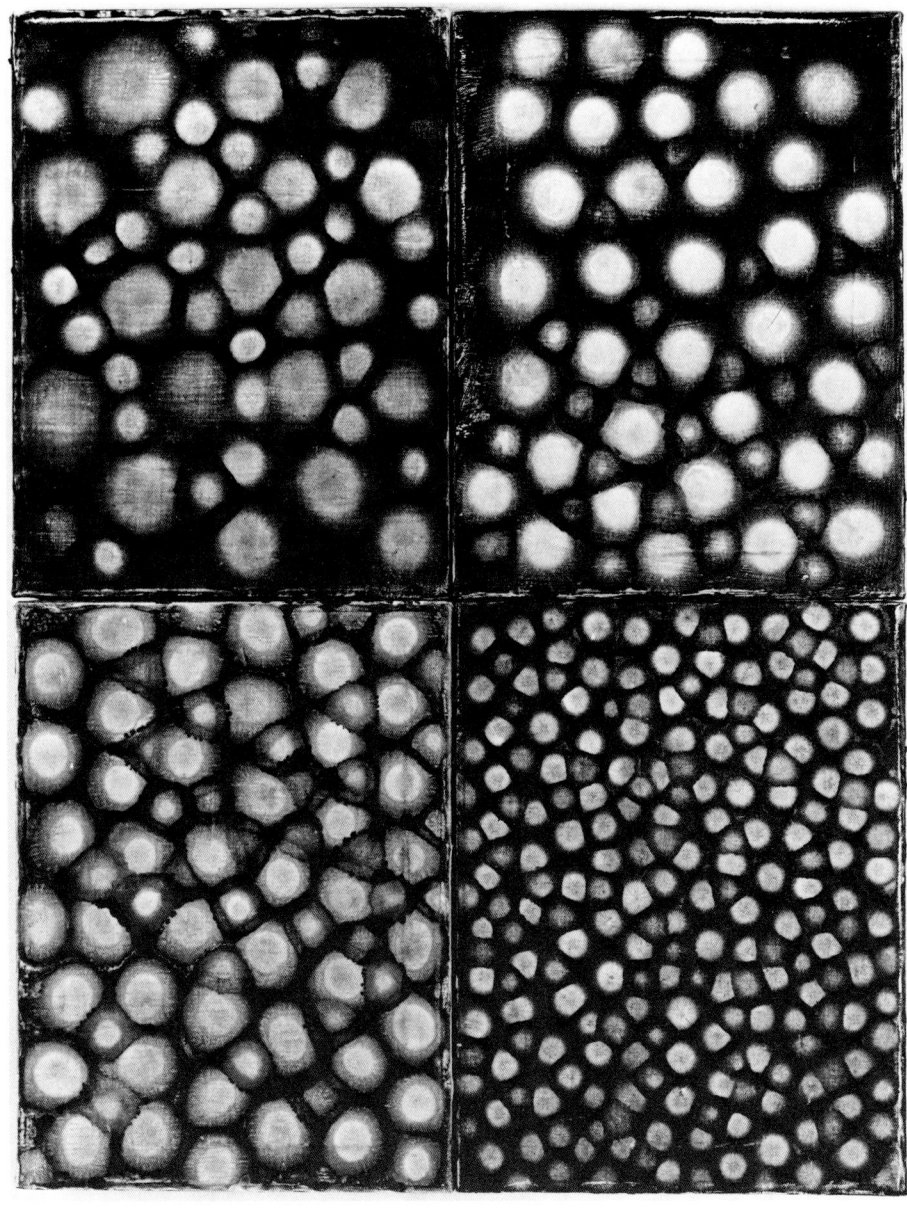

KATHE BURKHART

I Don't Have AIDS, 1990
From the series,
Liz Taylor (New York Post cover)
Acrylic, modeling paste, and
fake fur on canvas
78 × 78 inches

Kathe Burkhart confronts the sensationalistic and mean-spirited portrayal of AIDS by tabloid journalists. In Burkhart's canvas, celebrity Elizabeth Taylor—an indefatigable fund-raiser for AmFar (the American Foundation for AIDS Research)—has been put in the position of denying that she is a PWA, as if unselfish concern were an unfathomable motive for her efforts.

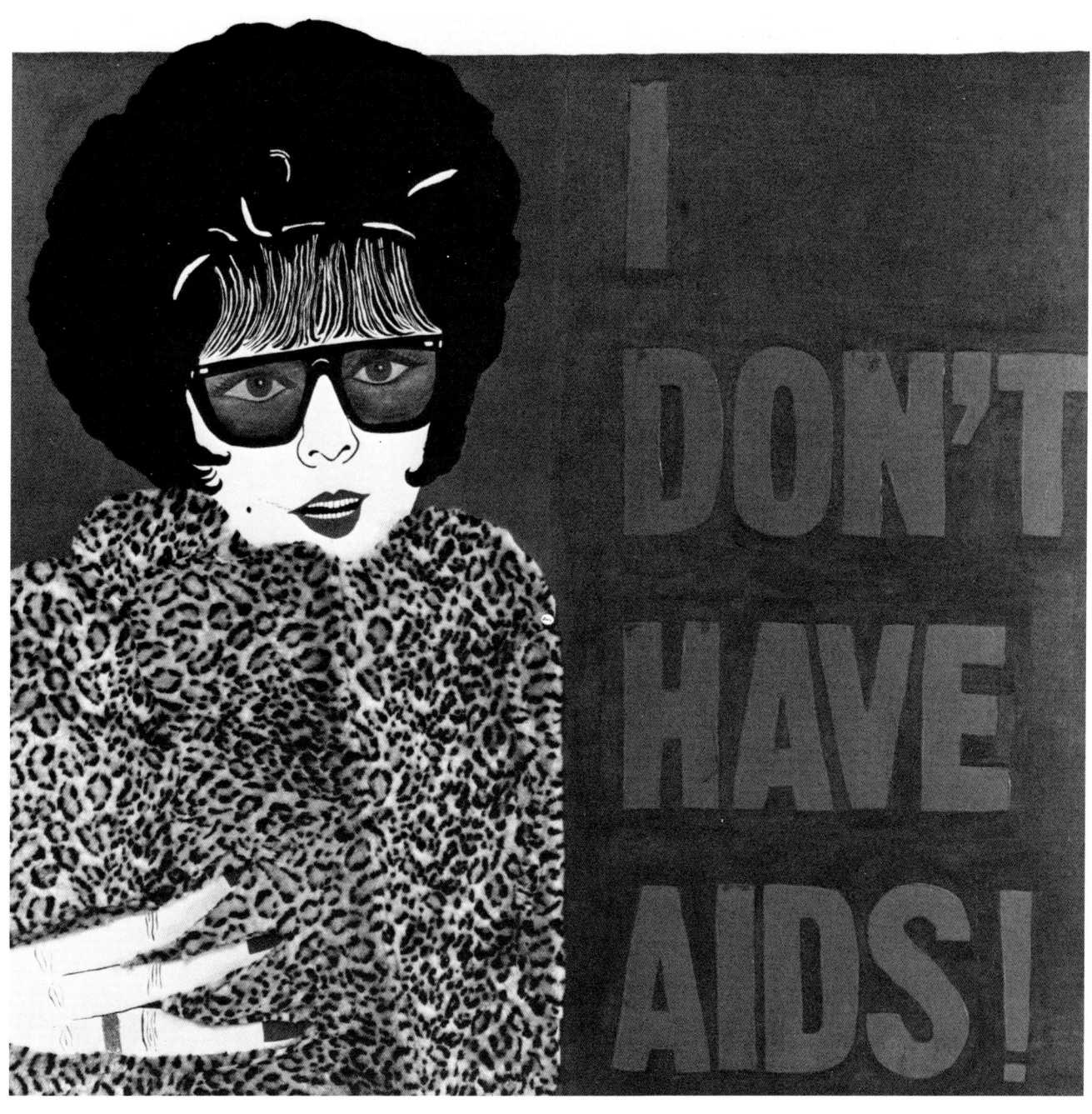

NANCY BURSON

Visualize This., 1991
Poster
18½ × 28½ inches

Nancy Burson's photo-microscopic images of healthy and HIV-infected T-cells have been put to dual purposes—as an artwork for in-gallery viewing, and as a street-sited object of visualization for PWAs. The poster—which appeared on New York walls in the spring of 1991—raised political issues, as so many AIDS-art projects do.

Some observers thought that the work placed responsibility for AIDS on PWAs, rather than on the slow-to-respond governmental and scientific establishments. Others supported Burson's project, believing that PWAs might partake of a range of treatments and activities—from holistic medicine to demonstrating in the streets.

Burson herself observed that "some HIV-infected people respond better than others to their condition or treatment and we don't know why." She began making visualization pieces in 1986 when her mother and best friend were terminally ill with cancer. "Visualization can be an empowering tool," she noted. "But no one should let the government off the hook."

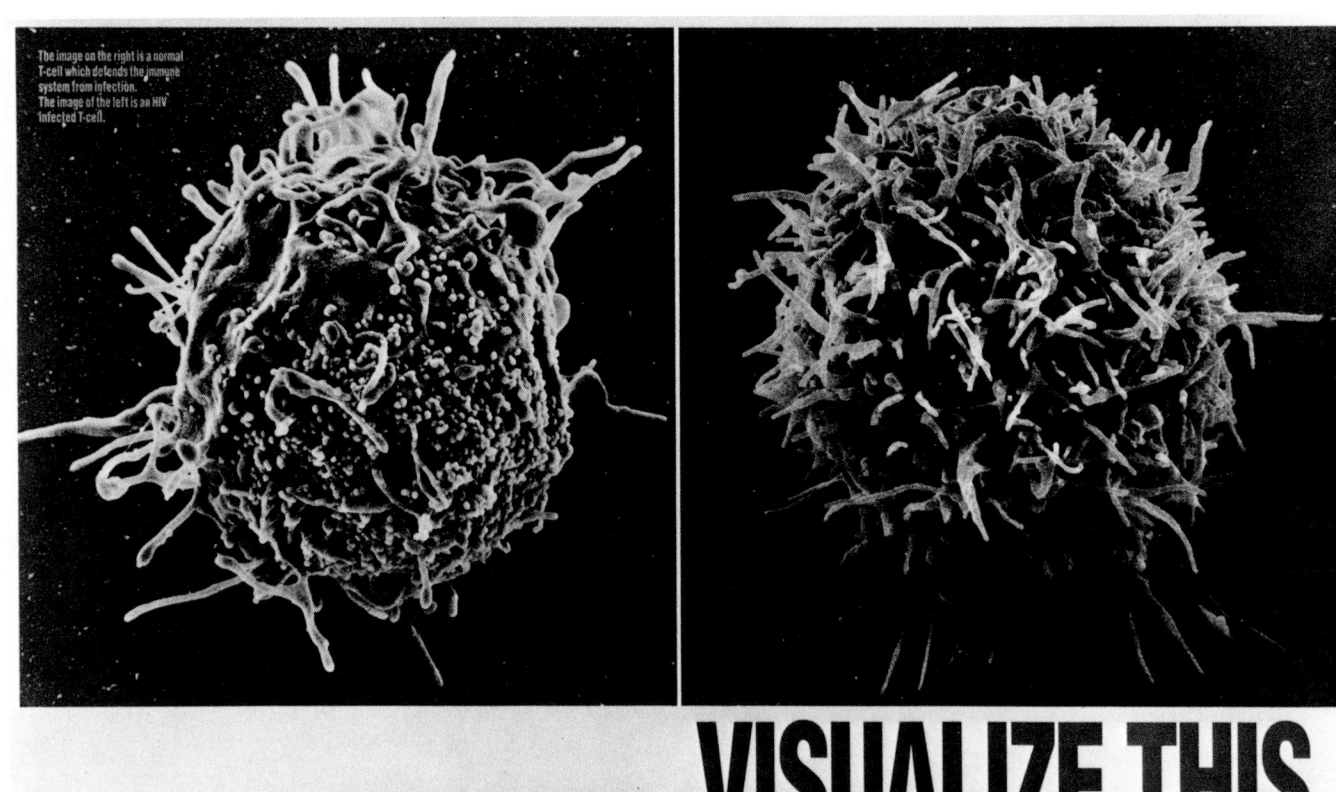

STEVEN EVANS

Composition in Pink, Black, and White (variation), 1986
Gelatin silver prints and latex and oil paint on masonite and wood
60½ × 68 inches overall

Steven Evans couples photographs of World War II Nazi concentration camps—in which homosexuals were imprisoned because of their sexual orientation and forced to wear pink triangles as identifying badges—with images from contemporary gay porno films. The geometric configuration of Evans's meditation on sexuality alludes to constructivism and evokes the rationale for that utopian approach to art, as well as Hitler's maniacal 'logic' in plotting the extermination of entire populations in order to 'purify' Aryan society.

Produced in 1986, Evans's work also refers to the then-current discussions of quarantining PWAs (as has been done in Cuba)—or to William F. Buckley's shocking suggestion that the HIV-infected be tattooed, as were concentration camp prisoners.

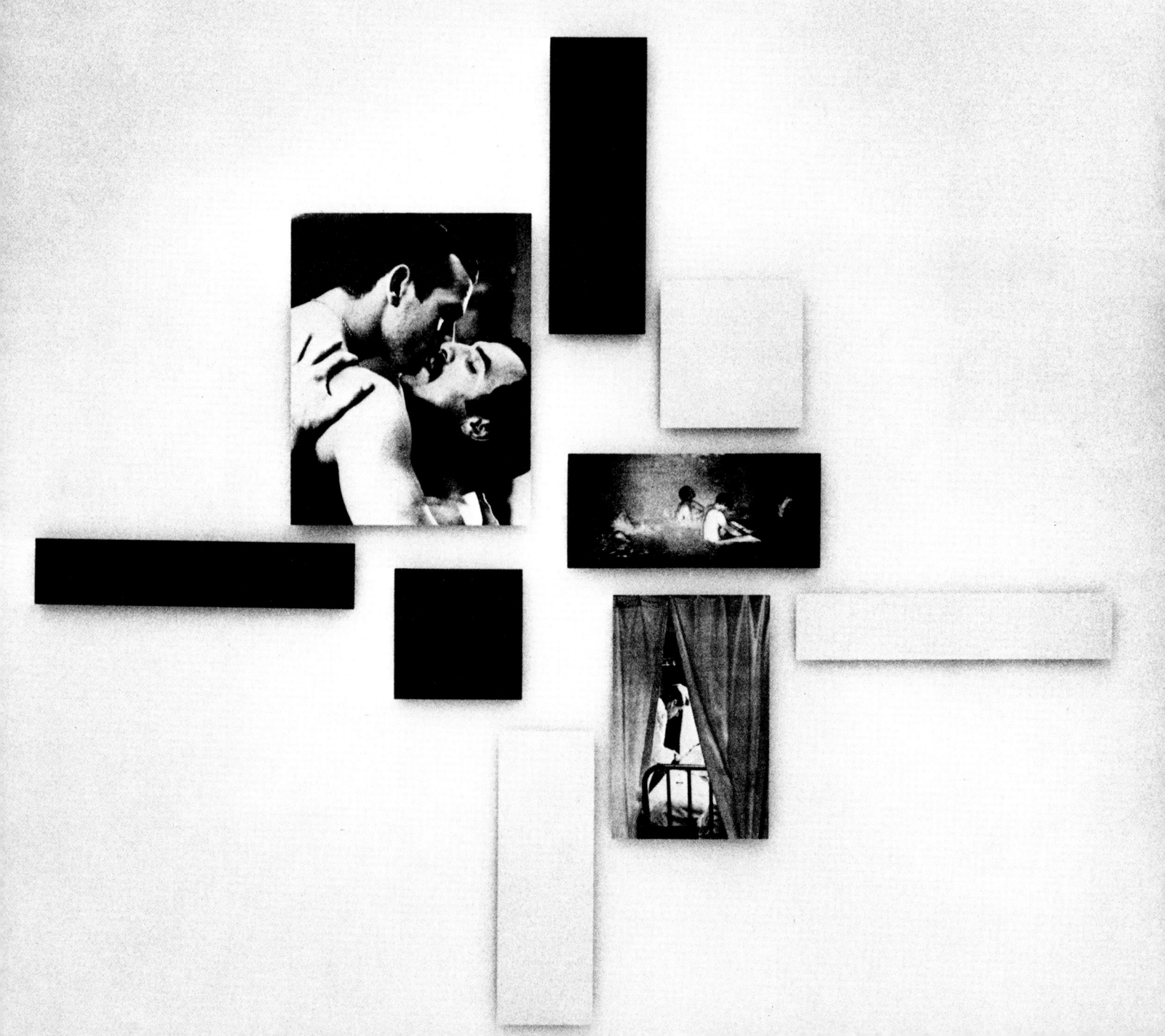

Composition in Pink, Black, and White (variation), 1986
Gelatin silver prints and latex and oil paint on masonite and wood
60½ × 68 inches overall

GENERAL IDEA

Imagevirus (Hamburg), 1989
1 of 5 Ektacolor RC prints
30 × 20 inches

The three-member Canadian collective, General Idea, has been producing artworks about AIDS since 1987. Their first AIDS works were based on Robert Indiana's iconic painting, *Love* (1966). By appropriating Indiana's format and altering its message, the artists hoped—and continue to hope—that their work will help "domesticate" the acronym for Acquired Immune Deficiency Syndrome and allow a more neutral discussion of AIDS to enter the discourse of daily life. These prints are documents of General Idea's street works which are pasted onto bus kiosks and billboards throughout the world.

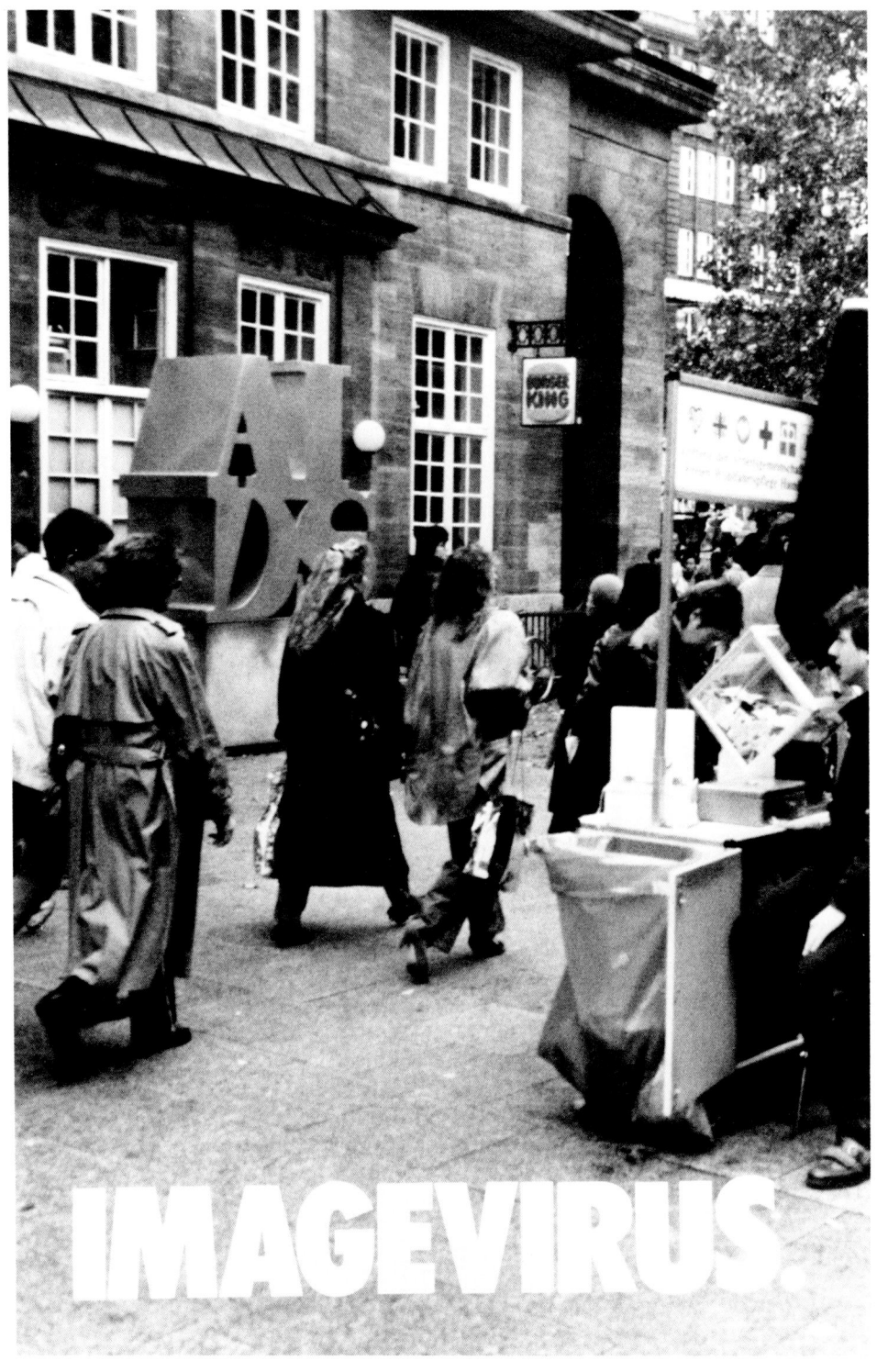

FELIX GONZALEZ-TORRES

Untitled, 1988
Framed photostat
10½ × 11¾ inches

Felix Gonzalez-Torres's untitled photostats evoke the value-laden "construction" of history—that is, the chaotic events and conditions that the media (or historians) order (or ignore), and then present, as sometimes conflicting versions of history. Patient Zero is the Canadian airline steward thought—by journalist Randy Shilts, author of the AIDS chronicle *And the Band Played On* (1987)—to have carried the HIV virus from Africa to North America.

Gonzalez-Torres is also a member of Group Material, the art-making collective that produced the AIDS Timeline, excerpted in the catalogue of this exhibition.

KEITH HARING

Untitled (Billboard Design), 1989
Photostat
8 × 10 inches

When Keith Haring died of AIDS-related causes in 1990, he was one of the world's best-known artists. Although references to AIDS appear infrequently in his paintings, Haring supported AIDS causes with unstinting generosity and zeal. Starting in 1988, he donated t-shirt and poster designs, as well as the sculpture, *Totem*, to ACT UP. During the same month, at Pasadena's Art Center College of Design, Haring painted a 24-by-10-foot mural depicting viral images. This was his contribution to the first Day Without Art—a national day of action and mourning organized by Visual AIDS in response to the AIDS crisis.

For Art Against AIDS' "On the Road" project, realized in San Francisco in 1989, Haring produced the billboard design that appears in this exhibition. He produced his *Silence=Death* print for ACT UP the same year. The pink triangle refers to the identifying badge worn by homosexuals incarcerated in Hitler's concentration camps. Gay liberationists had inverted the triangle in the 1970s; in 1986, the Silence=Death Project, a New York group, appropriated the Nazi's upright triangle for this logo-symbol that has become an internationally known signifier of AIDS activism.

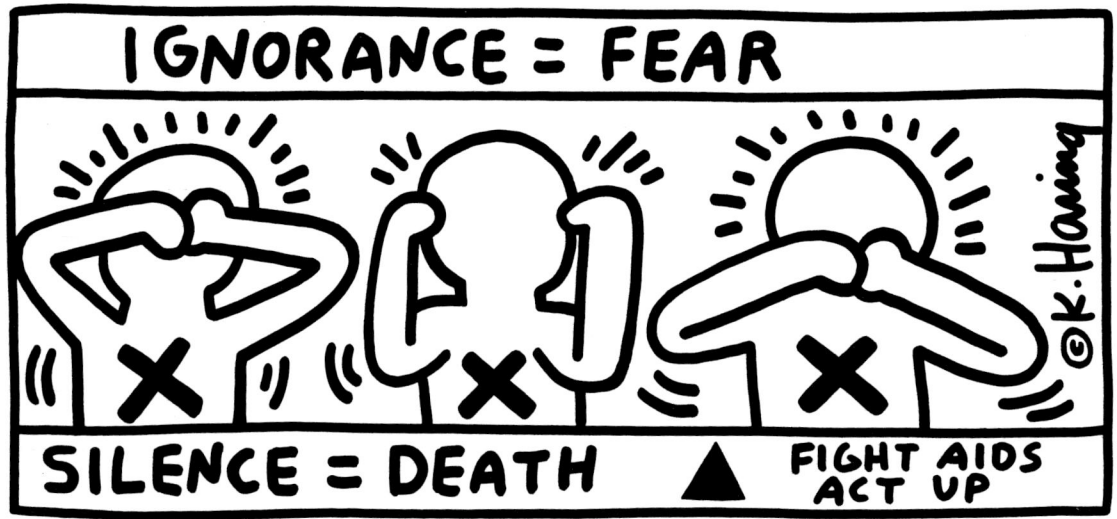

ADRIAN KELLARD

The Promise/I Will Never Leave You, 1989
Carved wood with paint
75 × 45 × 2 inches

Adrian Kellard's work evokes medieval roadside shrines through its materials (roughly carved wood blocks that suggest the folkloric output of artisans) and its imagery—in this case, the legend of St. Christopher who ferried the infant Jesus across a turbulent river. The title, *The Promise/I Will Never Leave You*, reaffirms the artist's belief in divine mercy, especially for the seriously ill. Adrian Kellard died of complications from HIV infection in the fall of 1991.

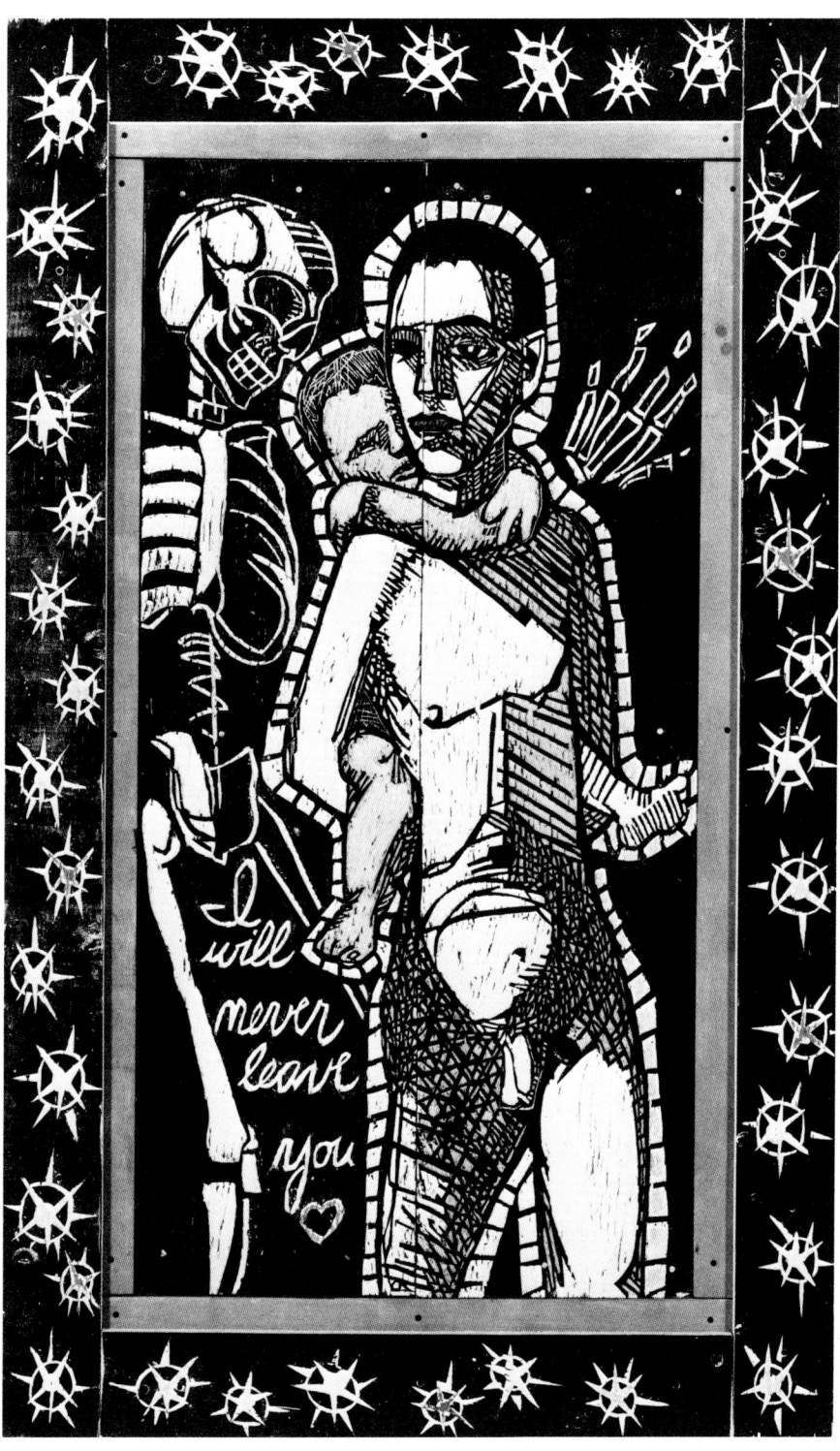

PETER KUNZ-OPFERSEI

1 page from *Book of Drawings* #2, 1987-88
Mixed media on paper, 39 pieces
9⅛ × 6⅜ inches each page

Peter Kunz-Opfersei, a Swiss-born artist who lived in New York, died of HIV-related causes in 1988. The exhibited sketchbooks that the artist produced in the last months of his illness are marked by a playful blend of healing images—shamans, magi, and sensuous ephebes.

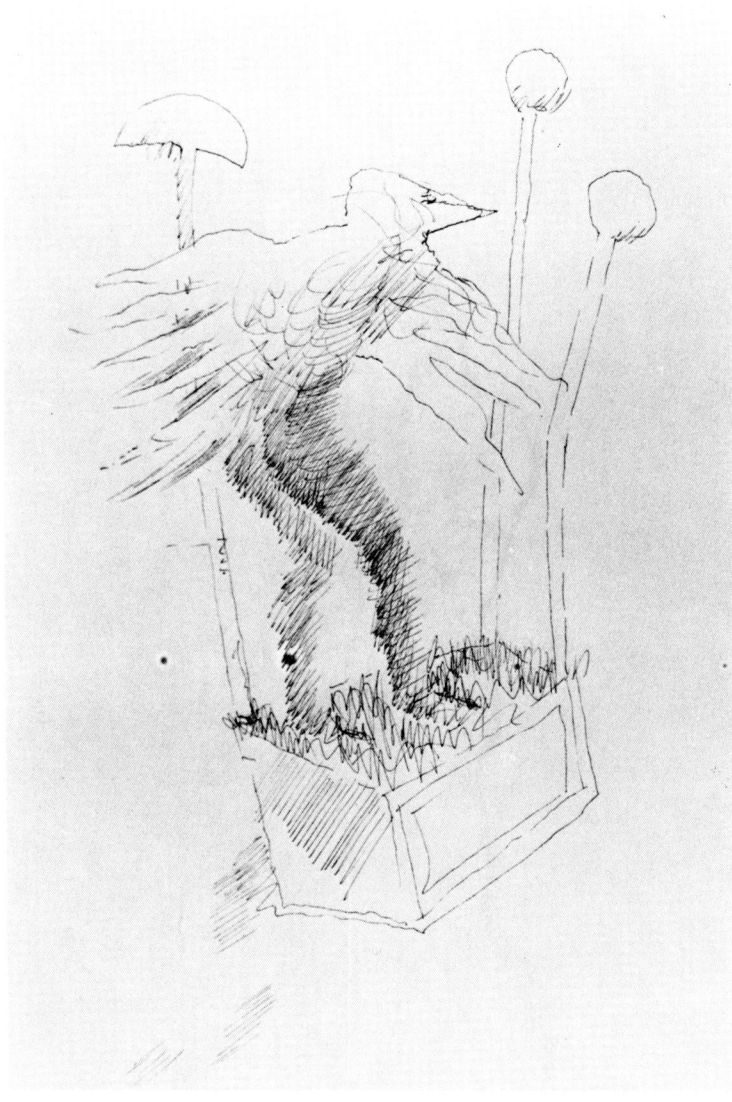

RUDY LEMCKE

Garden, 1988 (detail)
Architectural model for AIDS monument
½ scale model, 24 × 24 × 7 inches

Rudy Lemcke's vision of an AIDS memorial in San Francisco's Castro district is a meditative, Zen garden featuring a river of stones flowing over black granite, complemented by large bronzed boulders for seating. The memorial proved controversial within San Francisco's gay community when city officials approved the proposal in 1988. Those opposed said that a memorial should await a cure for AIDS, and that the required $250,000 (to be raised privately) would be better spent on research or treatment. Lemcke responded that other memorials, including the NAMES Project Quilt, already existed and that funding for arts and urban renewal projects was not likely to be channeled toward health care.

In his words: "I certainly am in agreement that health care is the priority issue. But psychological health, spiritual health, and political health are also very real needs that must be acknowledged. The garden will help care for those needs. It will create a comforting place to express grief, a meditative place to experience hope, and a permanent place to celebrate our identity." His fund-raising efforts are currently on hold.

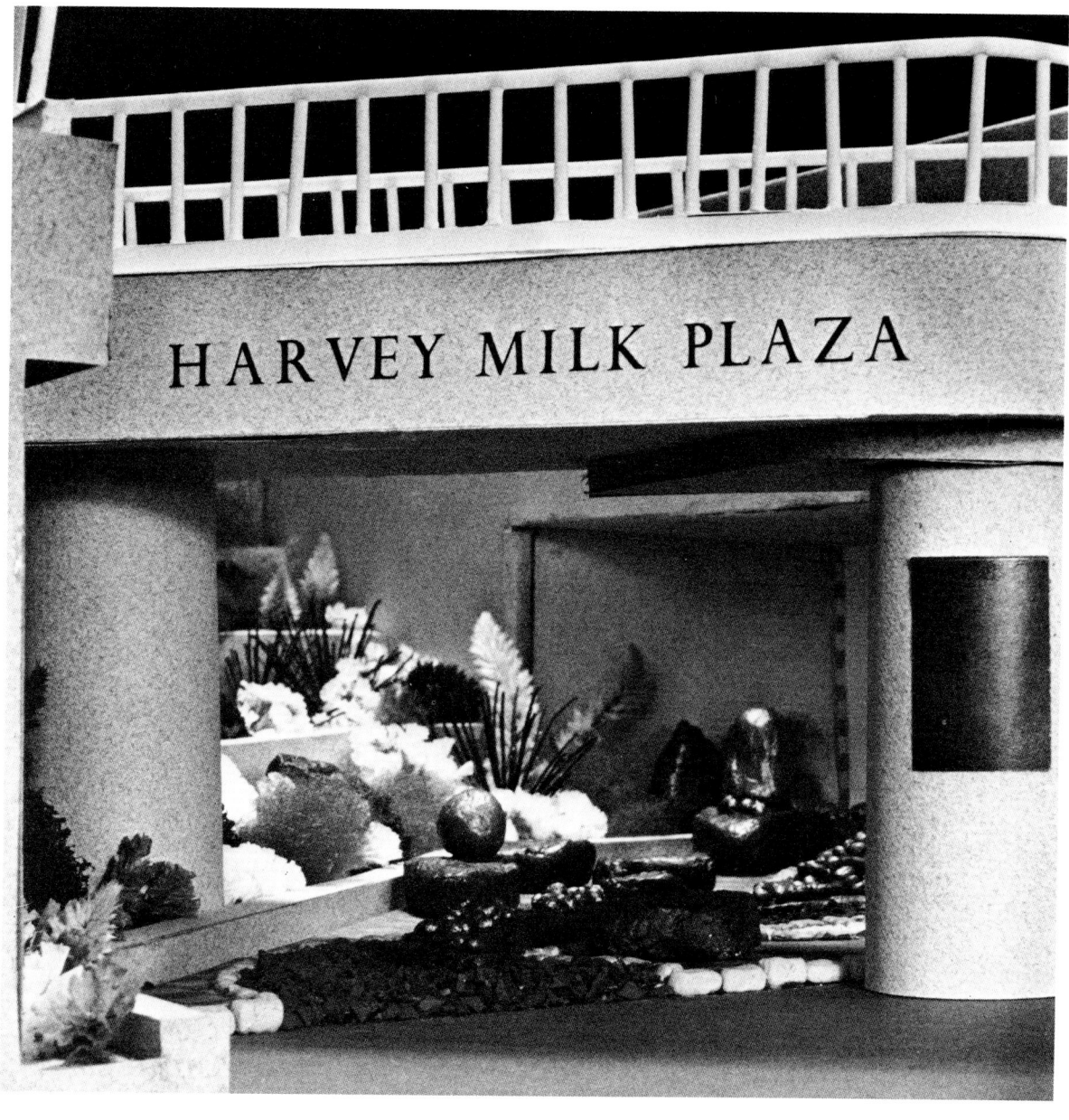

ROBERT MAPPLETHORPE

Self-Portrait, 1988
Gelatin silver print
24 × 20 inches
©1988, The Estate of
Robert Mapplethorpe

This iconic image, complete with *memento mori*, is the last of an ongoing series of self-portraits by Robert Mapplethorpe—the artist most associated in the public mind with homosexuality and AIDS. (Mapplethorpe died of HIV-related causes in 1989.) *The Perfect Moment*, a retrospective exhibition of Mapplethorpe's frank images of his own—and others'—sexual practices, helped catalyze the continuing debate about the public funding of art. When Washington, D.C.'s Corcoran Gallery of Art cancelled the show just prior to its opening in 1989, the art community enacted a virtual boycott of the museum. In 1990, Dennis Barrie, director of Cincinnati's Contemporary Arts Center, was charged with violating obscenity laws in presenting the exhibition. A jury acquitted him.

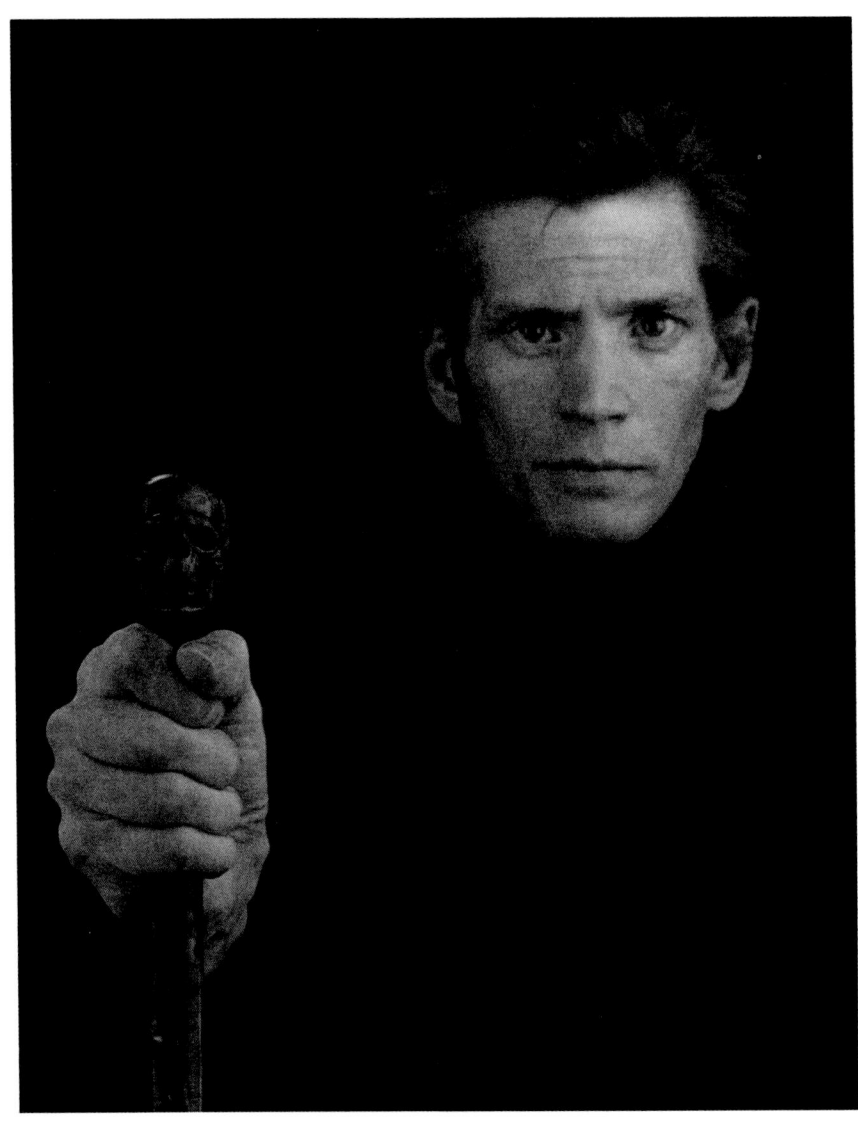

PAUL MARCUS

Maze of AIDS, 1989
Oil on wood
72 × 96 inches

Paul Marcus's woodblock chronicles the adult life of Yvonne, a young Hispanic woman with AIDS who lived with her son in the Bronx. The maze evokes the dead-end social conditions of impoverished urban ghettoes that essentially promote drug use and exposure to HIV-infection because of their lack of social services, decent housing, and employment opportunities.

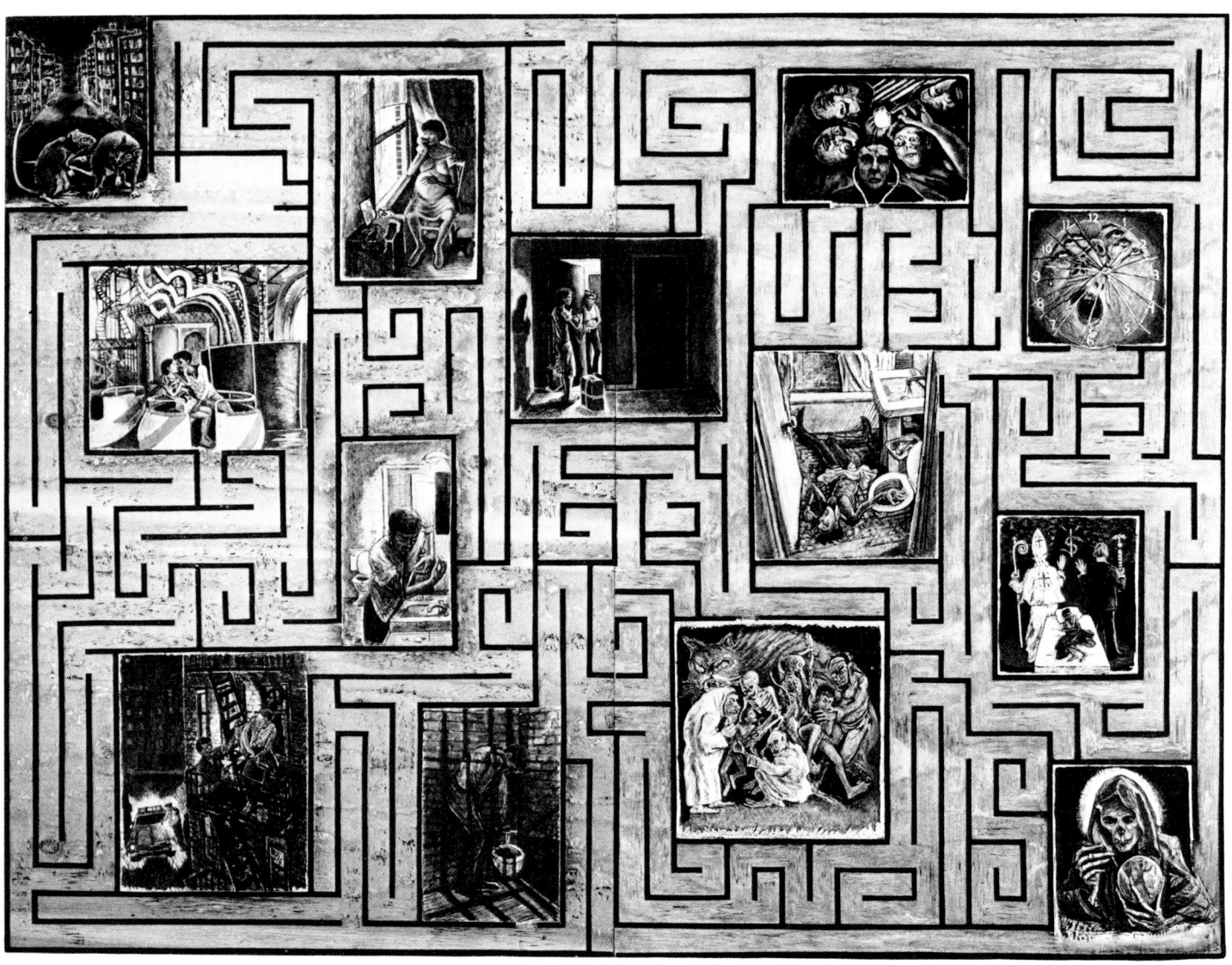

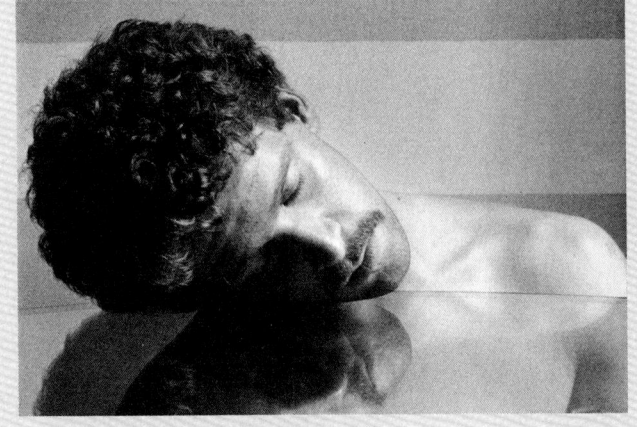

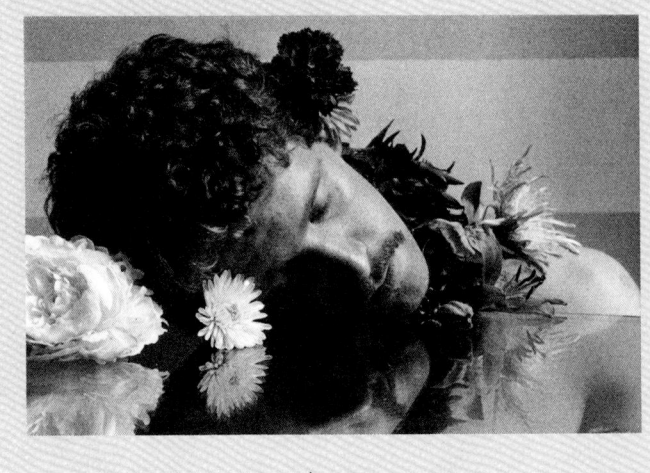

DUANE MICHALS

The Dream of Flowers, 1986
Gelatin silver prints
5 × 7 inches each

Duane Michals poetically evokes grief in this elegy to lives tragically shortened by HIV illness. Michals envisions death as a gradual fading away rather than an abrupt end, and he symbolizes this poignantly by means of the expanding veil of flowers that envelops the head of his model.

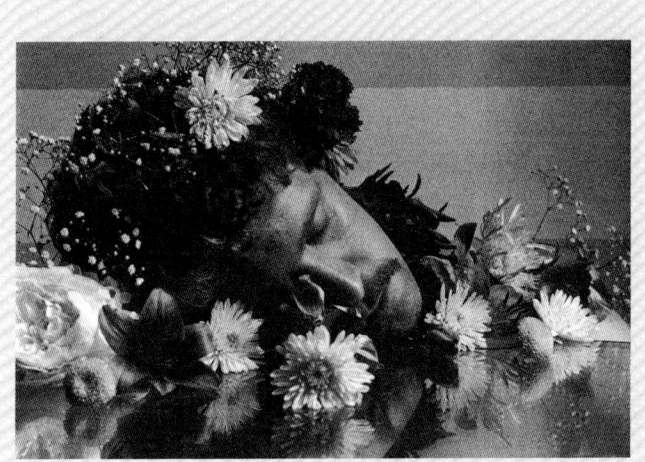
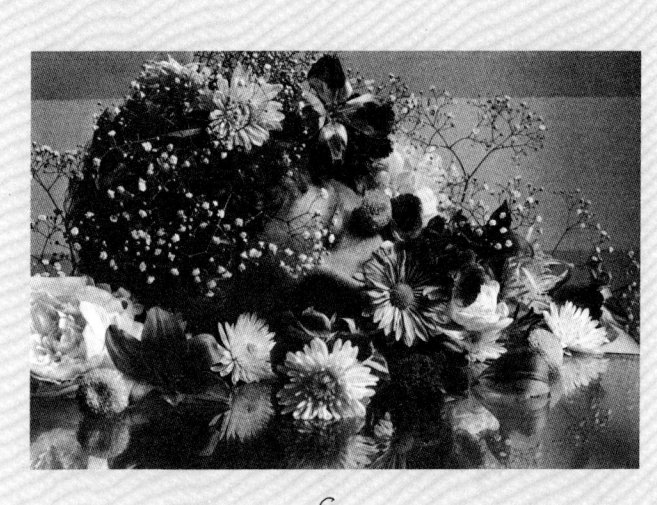

DONALD MOFFETT

Call the White House, 1990
Back-lit Ciba-transparency
40 × 60 × 7 inches

Donald Moffett—an AIDS activist and member of Gran Fury—refers in this work to the federal government's mismanagement of the AIDS crisis. The government's own Watkins Commission issued a 1988 report harshly critical of the continuing incoherence and short-sightedness of federal AIDS policies.

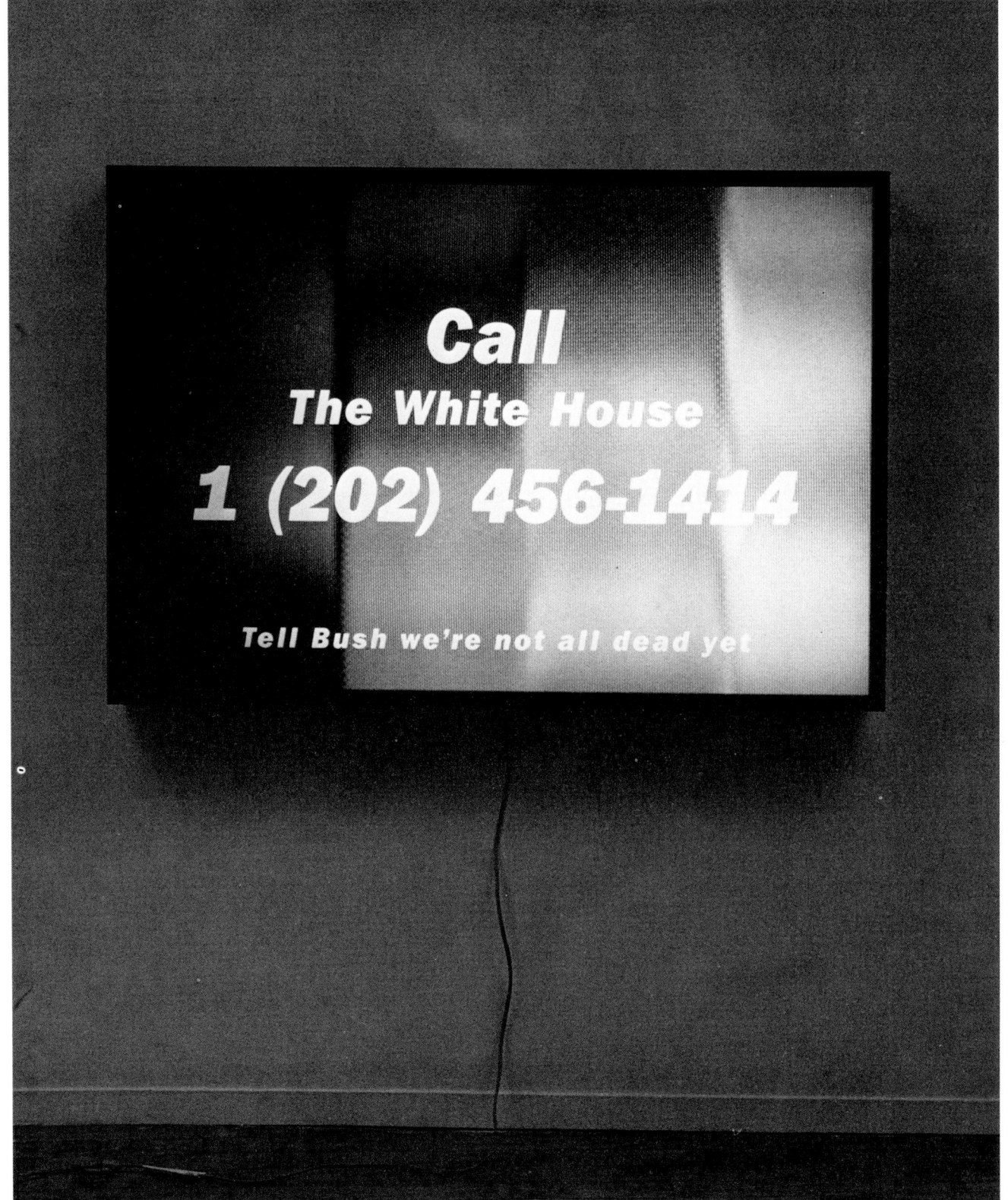

FRANK MOORE

Bubble Bath, 1990
Oil on canvas with mixed media
83½ × 99½ inches

Frank Moore, an artist and set designer, painted this work following his now deceased lover's AIDS diagnosis. In highly personal fashion, Moore couples his ecological and AIDS-related concerns in a dense web of imagery that includes references to circulation systems, metastasis, information, loss, waste, stigmatization, anal- and safer-sex.

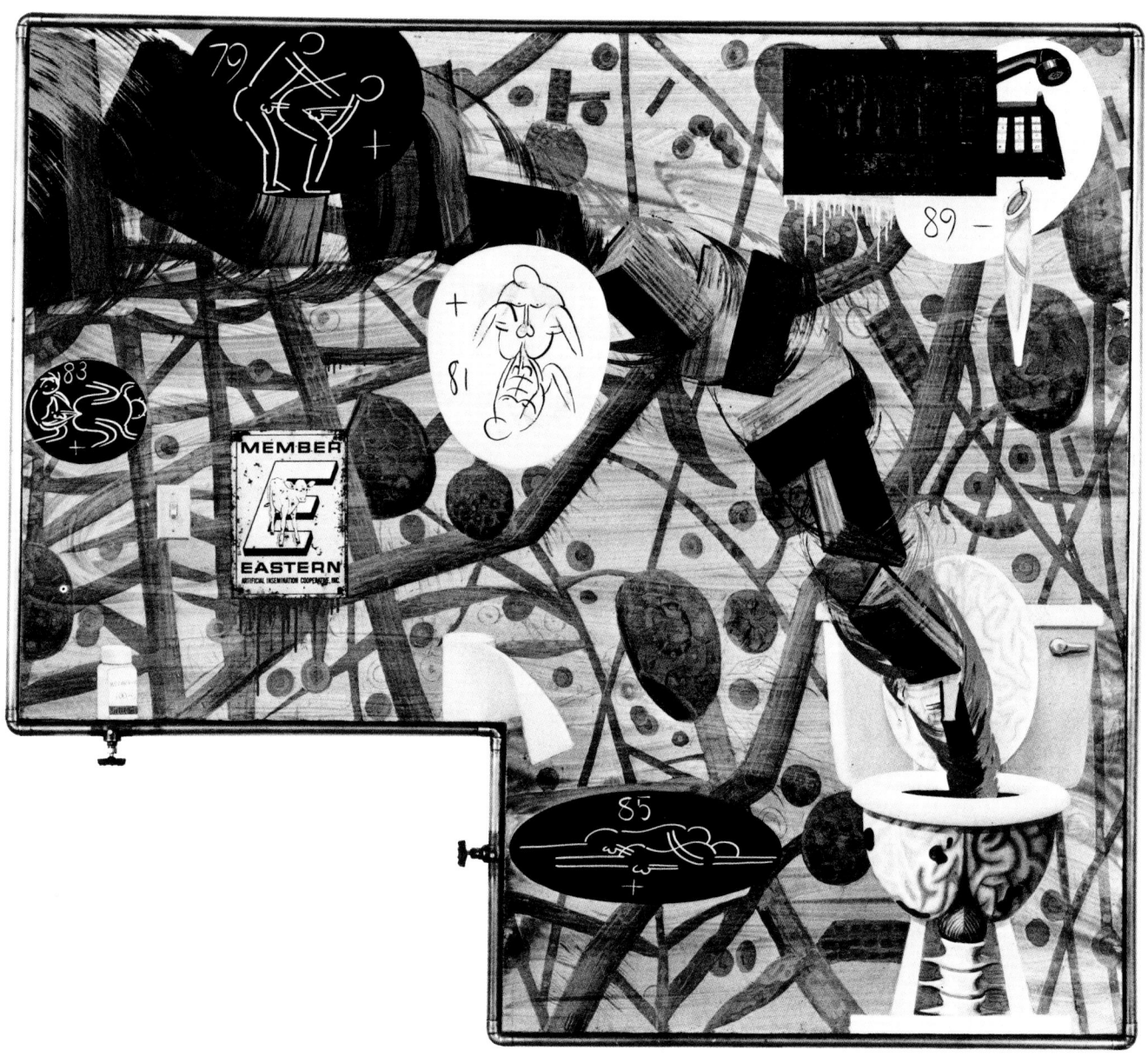

ELLEN B. NEIPRIS

ACT UP, Republican National Convention (New Orleans), 1988
Gelatin silver print
11 × 14 inches

"After a half dozen arrests as a member of ACT UP for the past four years, I continue to struggle with myself. Is documenting this crisis—using my camera as my political voice—enough? Or do I have to put my body on the line to really make a difference? Working as a professional photojournalist now, I still struggle to answer these questions and to decide what my role is in this community and in this crisis."

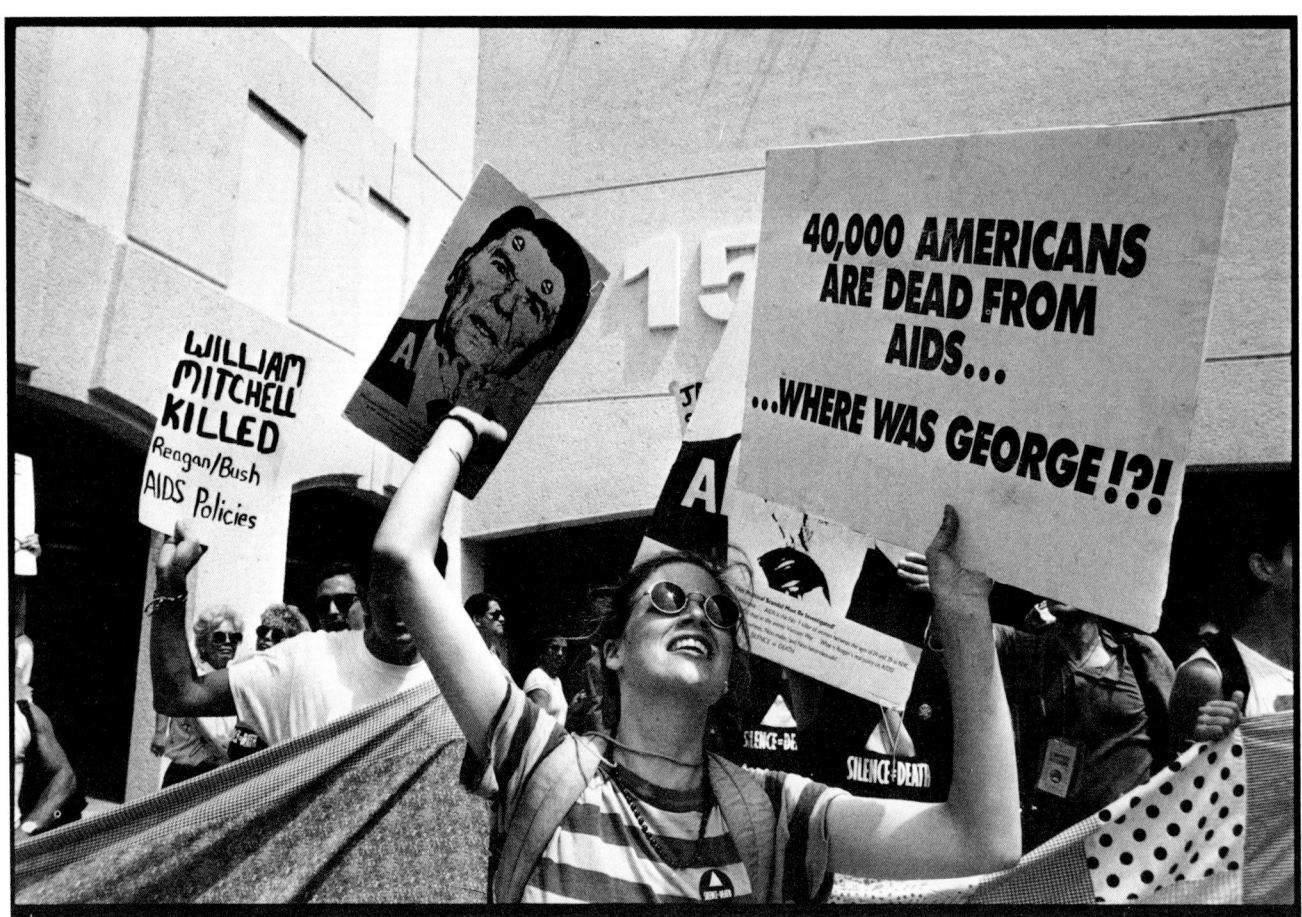

DIANE NEUMAIER

Untitled, 1988
From the series,
Street Graphic Interventions
Black-and-white resin-coated print
16 × 20 inches

Diane Neumaier's photographs are documents of the Metropolitan Health Association's February 1988 action in the New York subway. The guerrilla group plastered bilingual how-to information about using condoms and cleaning drug 'works' onto subway ad placards. Their interventions were removed within twelve hours, but Neumaier's images remain.

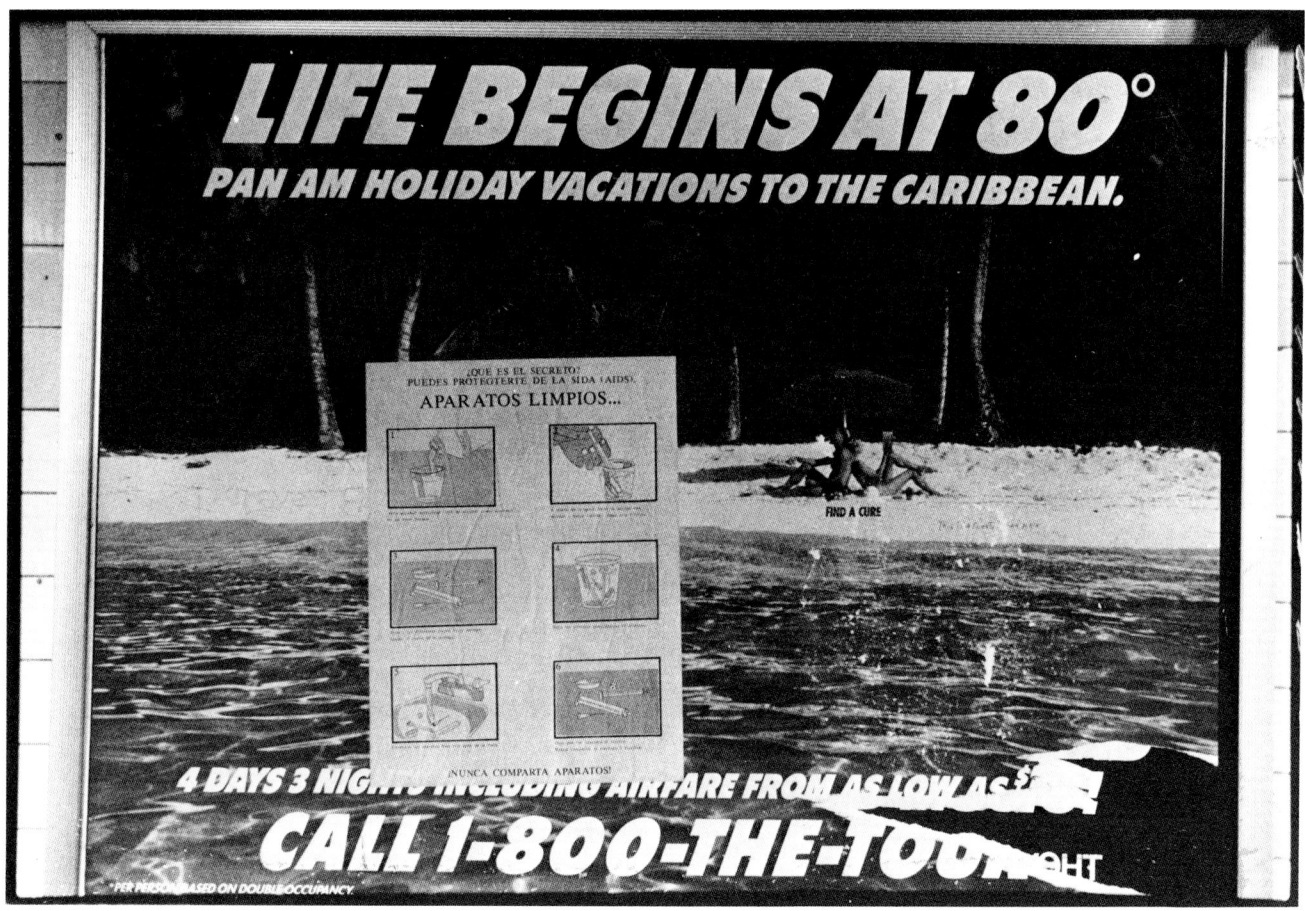

NICHOLAS AND BEBE NIXON

Laverne Colebut, 1988–89
8 gelatin silver prints and text
8 × 10 inches each

The components of Nicholas Nixon's serial portraits of PWAs were shot at numerous regular intervals; six to twelve images were culled for each 'portrait'. Nixon's pictures, some of the first photo-portraits of PWAs exhibited at a major museum, appeared at a moment when representations of AIDS were largely limited to horrific images from the mainstream media. At his Museum of Modern Art retrospective exhibition in 1988, ACT UP members distributed leaflets criticizing the work for its lack of social context and calling for positive images of PWAs who are "vibrant, sexy, loving, and acting up." Admirers of Nixon's work, on the other hand, applaud what they regard as the work's power and unshrinking realism.

The interview exhibited in conjunction with the pictures comes from *People With AIDS*, a book of photos and interview texts published in 1991 by Nixon and science journalist Bebe Nixon. Bebe Nixon has been conducting interviews with PWAs and their loved ones since 1987, when the project began.

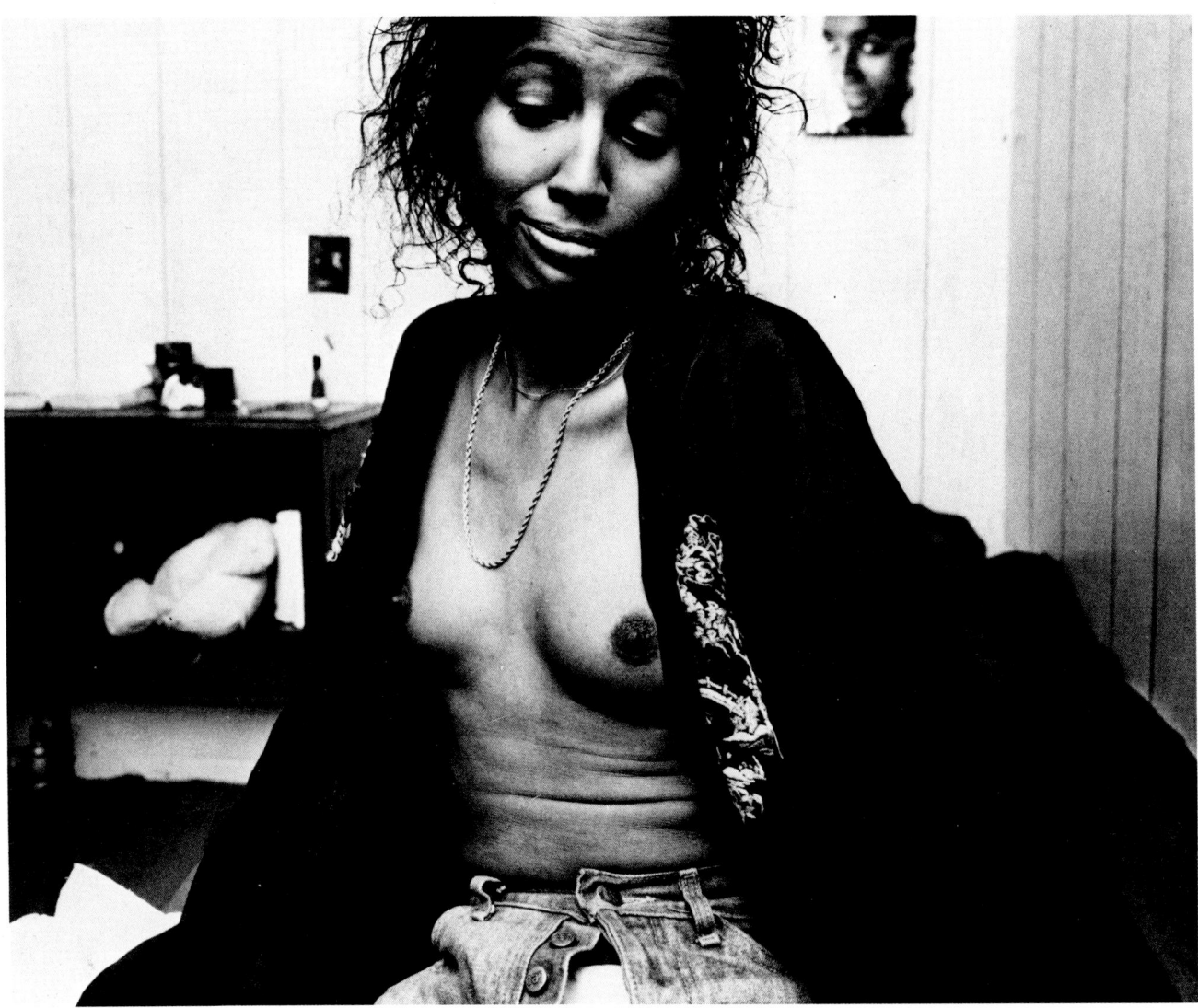

NICHOLAS NIXON *Laverne Colebut*, Providence, RI, October, 1988.

GYPSY RAY

Zenobia and Jon, 1986
Gelatin silver print and text
20 × 16 inches

Gypsy Ray's photographic portraits give a human face to PWAs and to frequently overburdened care-givers—volunteers, doctors, and loved ones—in the AIDS community. By insetting their typed or handwritten commentary directly onto the mats of her prints, she also provides her subjects with voices. The viewpoints of PWAs have frequently been ignored in the homophobic, political climate that has sanctioned the transformation of AIDS from a public health matter into an acrimonious debate about morality. A legacy of the AIDS crisis is likely to be the militance of the unwell—a phenomenon already apparent among women with breast cancer—in lobbying for themselves. In the case of PWAs, this has been accomplished through organizations such as the PWA Coalition.

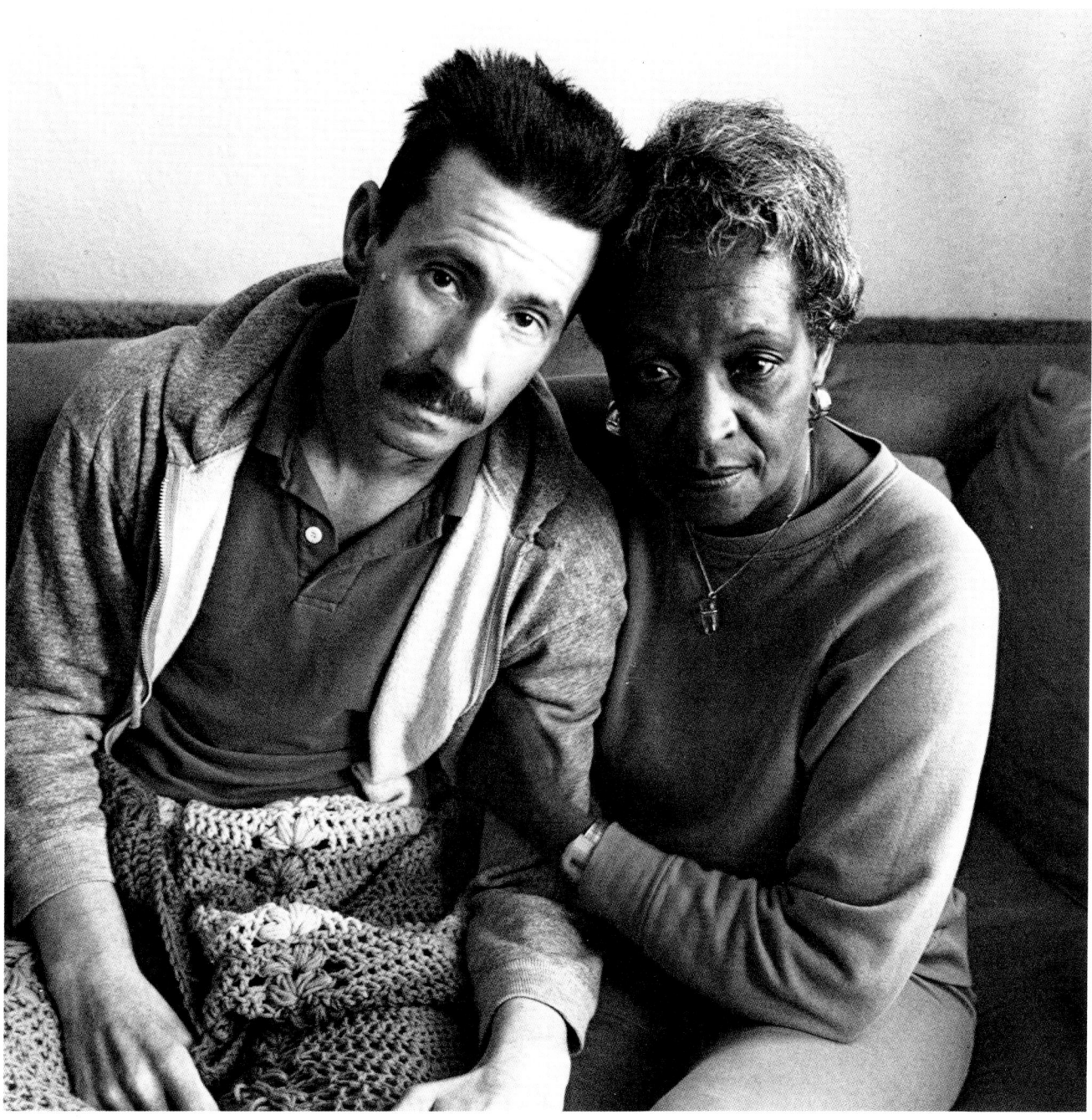

ROD RHODES

Stations of the Cross X, Stripping of Christ, 1988
Wood, glass, and felt
26 × 26 × 6¾ inches

In his *Stations of the Cross* series, Rod Rhodes coupled traditional Christian imagery and AIDS-related autobiography (he died of AIDS-related causes in 1989). The fourteen-work series of cruciform-shaped, glass-fronted tableaux culminates in the entombment. *Stations of the Cross X, Stripping of Christ* refers to the humiliating moment just before the mocking of Christ. For this rather abstract box, Rhodes removes himself and evokes Christ through the antlers, a recurring symbol in the series.

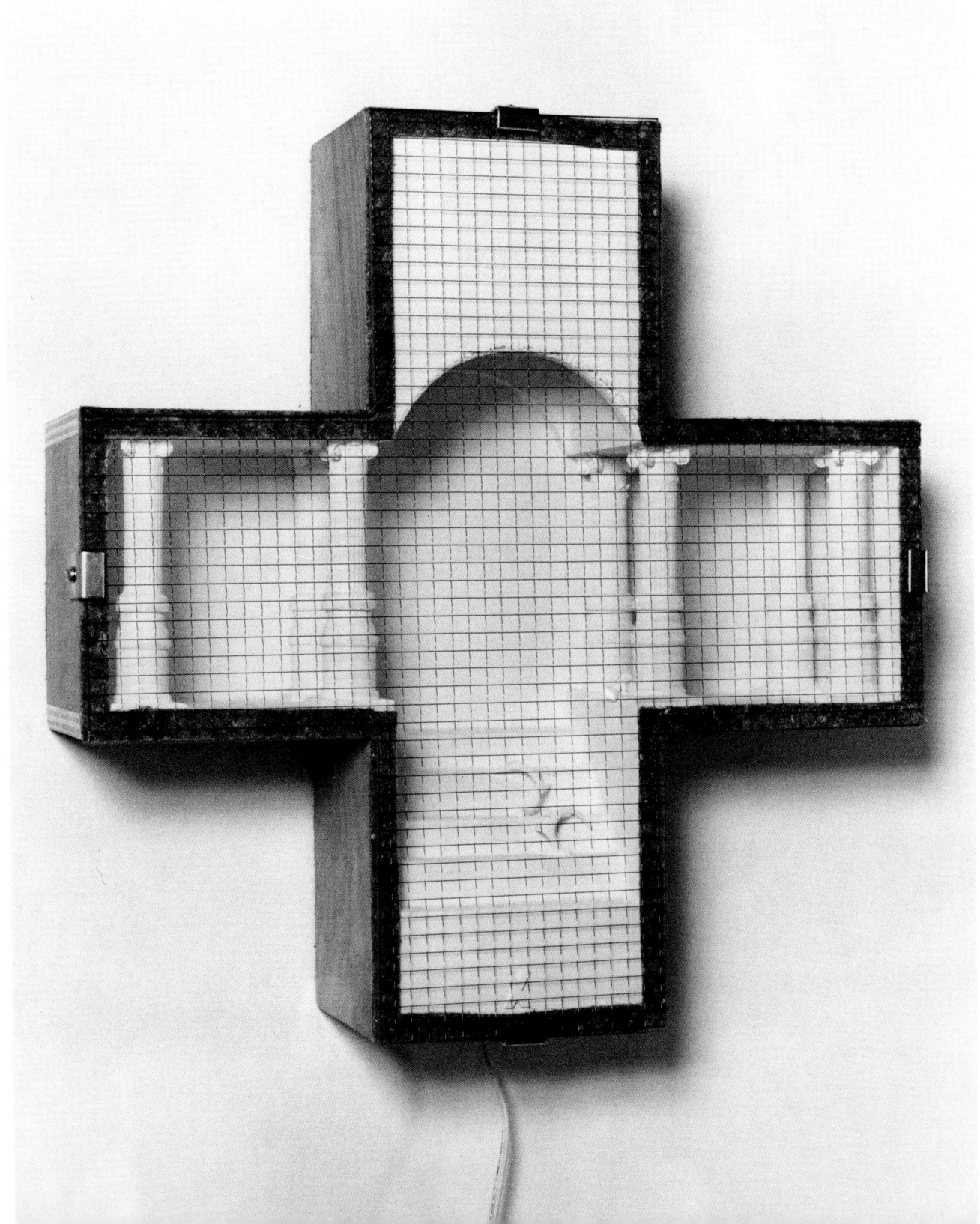

JANE ROSETT

Untitled, 1990
From the series, *Belle Glade, Florida*
Ektacolor RC print
16 × 20 inches

Jane Rosett's untitled photographs from the *Belle Glade, Florida* series were shot in the county with the highest incidence of HIV infection in the United States. A photojournalist and activist (she was one of the founders of New York's PWA Coalition and Community Research Initiative), Rosett frequently returns to this predominantly Haitian and Jamaican migrant farming community where, for lack of educational resources and social services, poverty and AIDS are being passed on to a new generation.

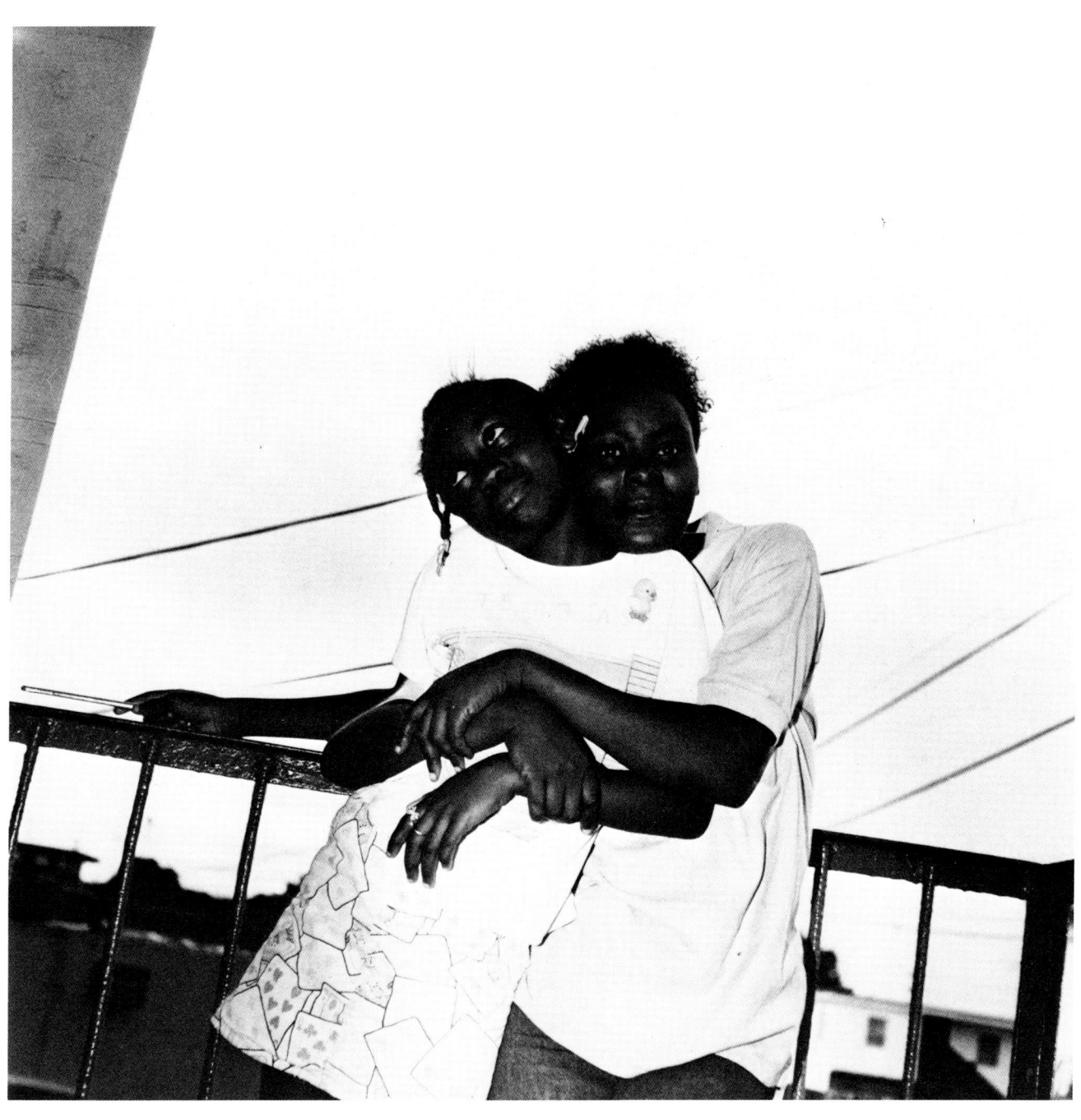

JOHN SAPP

Adam and I Finally Went to Key West, 1989
Charcoal on paper
60 × 84 inches

John Sapp's diaristic, sometimes humorous, drawings with texts are an insider's account of gay life in an era when HIV infection is no longer an out-of-the-ordinary phenomenon. Sapp's familiarity with AIDS may soon be the norm: the World Health Organization predicts 25 to 40 million cases of HIV infection world-wide by the end of the decade.

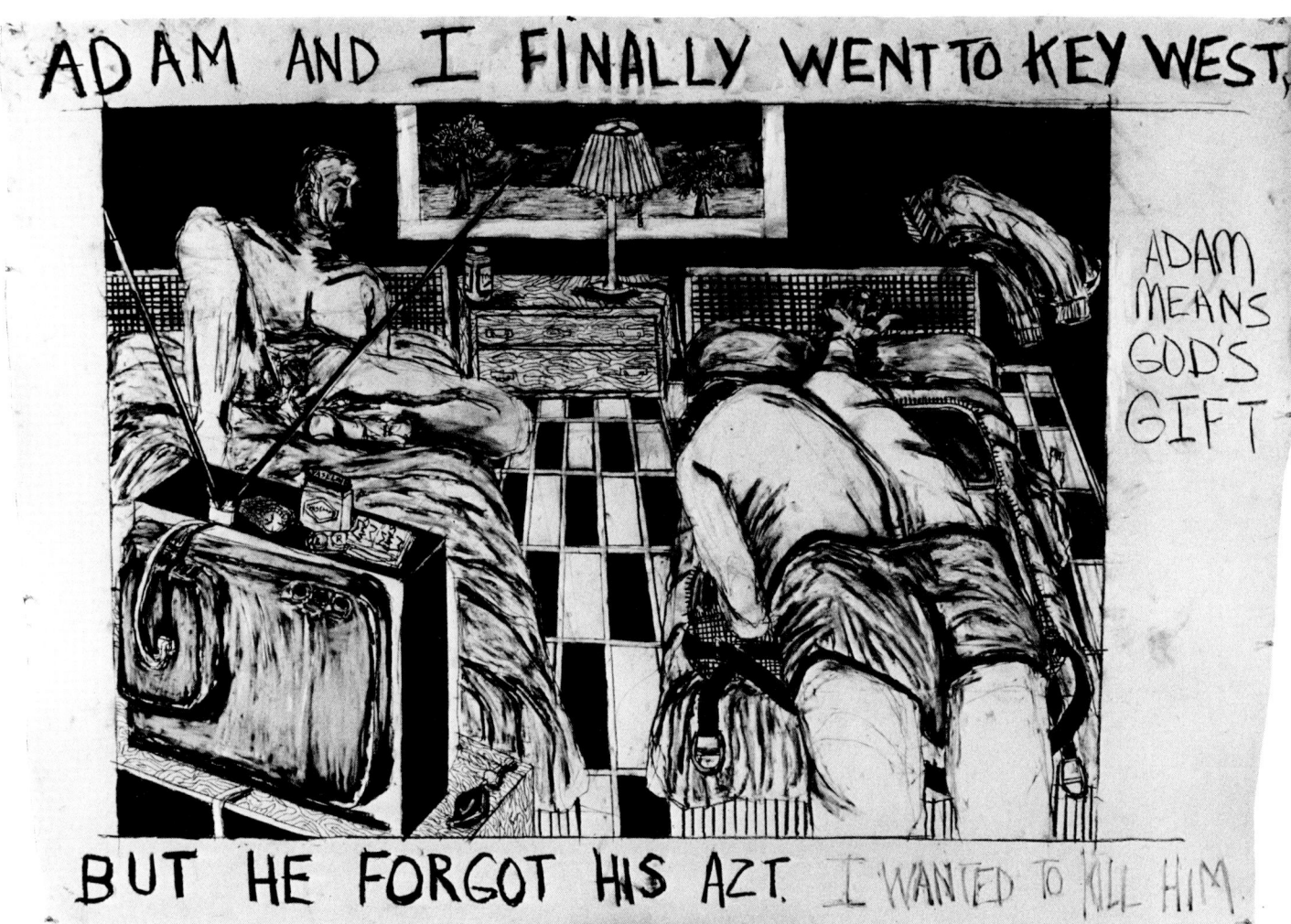

DUI SEID

Scum, 1989
Plastic, medical supplies, and framed text
96 × 72 × 6 inches

"As a home health care attendant for PWAs I began to understand that each person—PWA, family member, friend, or stranger—deals with AIDS in his [or her] own way.... This understanding informs my recent AIDS art in which people's different responses and associations to the disease are juxtaposed through the media of medical waste and words, allowing the viewer...to enter into an open discussion.... How can I prettify AIDS? That would be dishonest and exploitive.... Ironically, next year [1992] my not-very-pretty *AIDS/Words* series will probably be the first artworks overtly about AIDS to be exhibited in AIDS-phobic Japan."

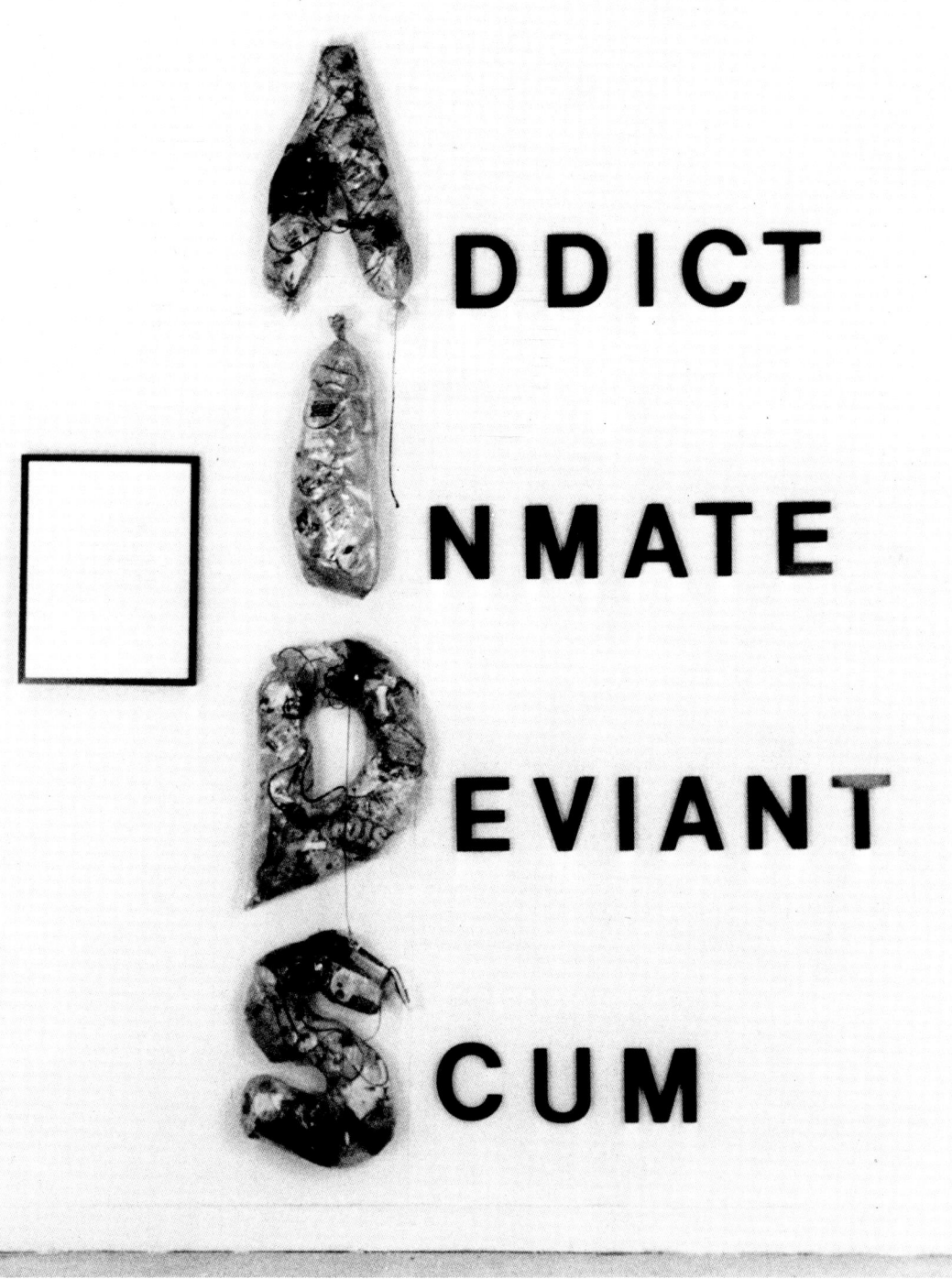

JO SHANE

*President's Choice
(This is a P.C. Product)*, 1991
Mixed-media installation
63¾ × 78 × 78 inches overall

Jo Shane's straightforward evocation of the apparent disposability of homosexual, non-white, or drug-using PWAs combines portraits of deceased PWAs and the aptly named "President's Choice" brand toilet paper. President Reagan did not mention the word "AIDS" in public until 1988.

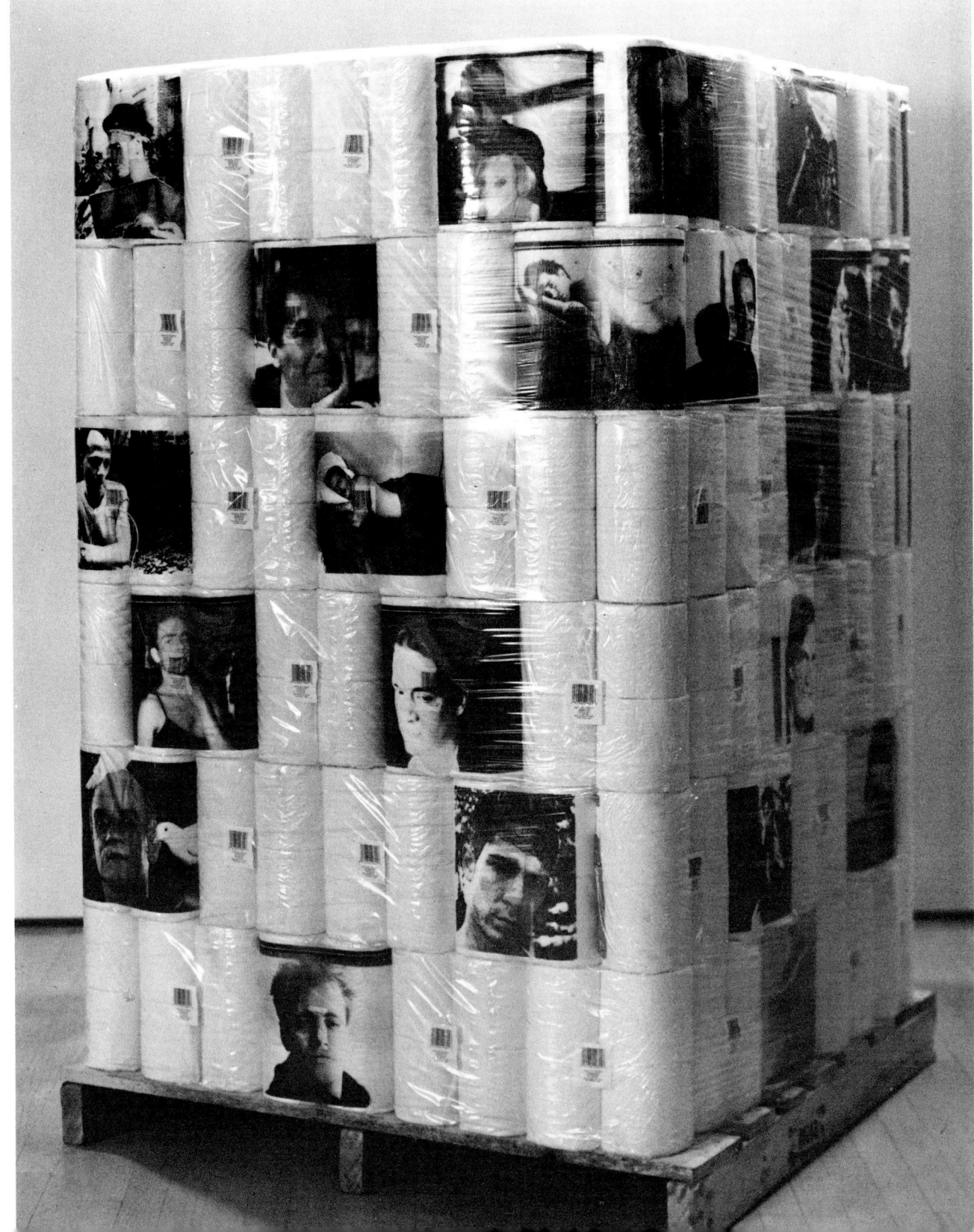

ROSALIND SOLOMON

Garden, New York, 1988
From the series,
Portraits in the Time of AIDS
Gelatin silver print
32 × 32 inches

In these works, Rosalind Solomon explores the meaning(s) of nature: the unnaturalness of parents confronting the prospect of a child's untimely death; the juxtaposition of a garden with evidence of the depicted PWA's immune-system breakdown in the form of Kaposi's Sarcoma (KS) lesions. KS, once a rare cancer, is now frequently found among male PWAs in the United States.

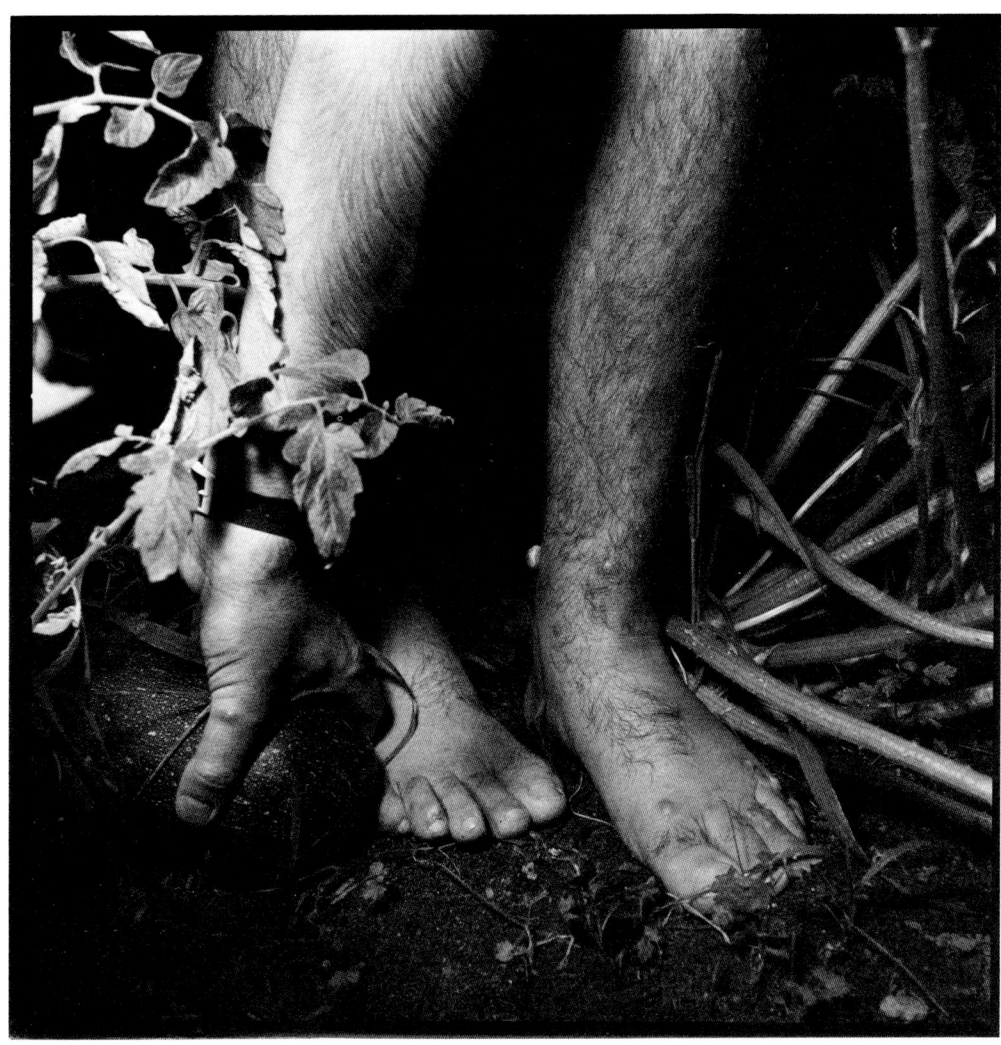

MASAMI TERAOKA

AIDS Series/Geisha and AIDS Nightmare, 1989–90
Watercolor on canvas
106¼ × 74 inches

Masami Teraoka's ongoing AIDS series was inspired by the death of a friend's child from AIDS complications. To viewers familiar with the Japanese Ukiyo-e prints that chronicled the "floating world" of the geisha-courtesan, the contemporary references to sexuality will be immediately apparent. Through their acrobatic actions, Teraoka's latter-day geishas advocate the use of condoms, as do the texts the artist renders directly on his paintings.

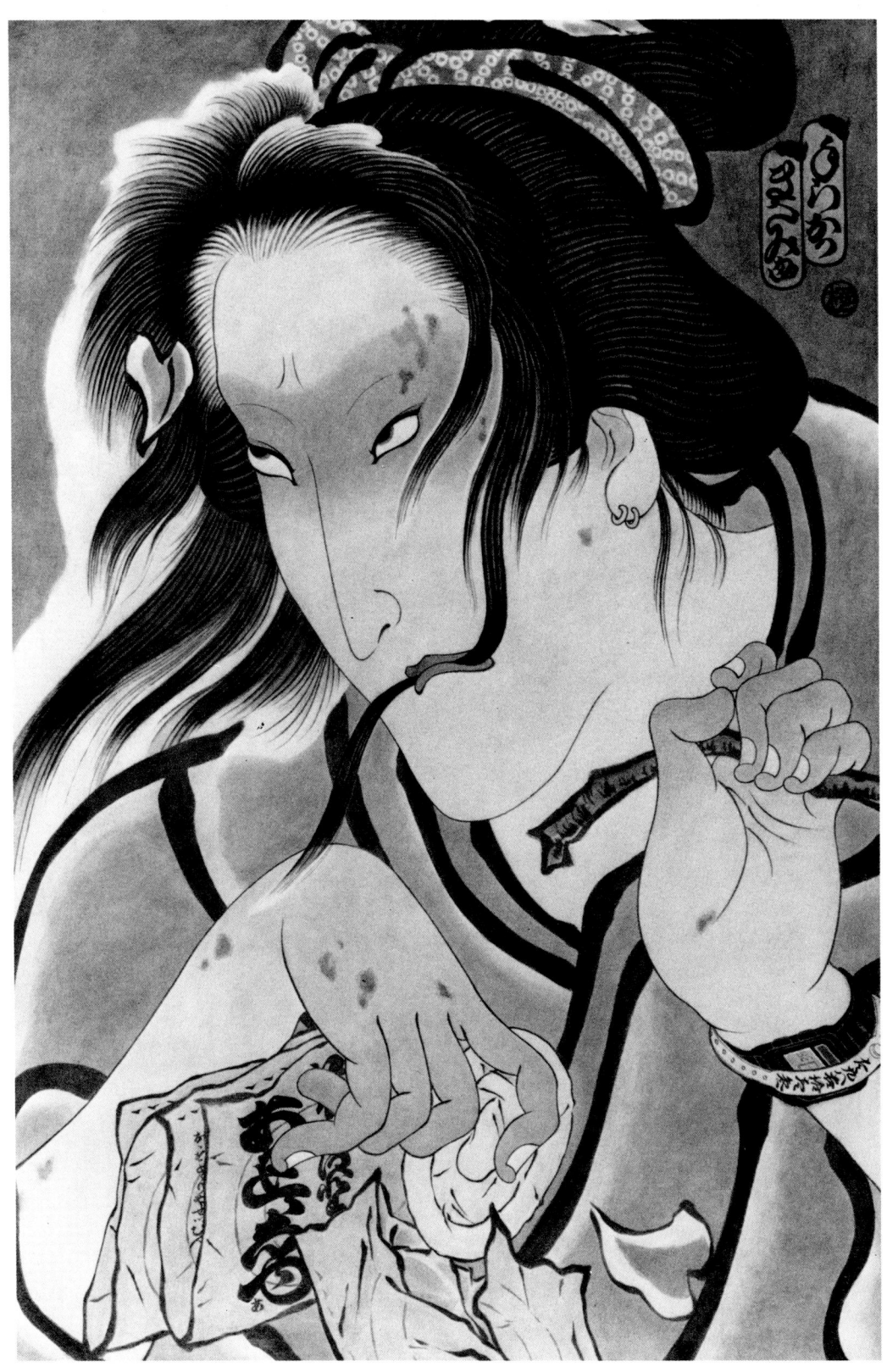

MAX (TORQUE) = DOUG [(BRUNO) HAMMETT]

Re-Circulate, 1990
From the series, *Sleeping Beauty*
Mixed-media sculpture
11 × 10 × 11 inches

Re-Circulate is part of the artist's *Sleeping Beauty* series. Fairy-tale reality implies that the longed-for vaccine might be the revitalizing equivalent of a prince's kiss. The once lethal nature of the encased material suggests an artifact or curio comparable to a scorpion embedded in resin.

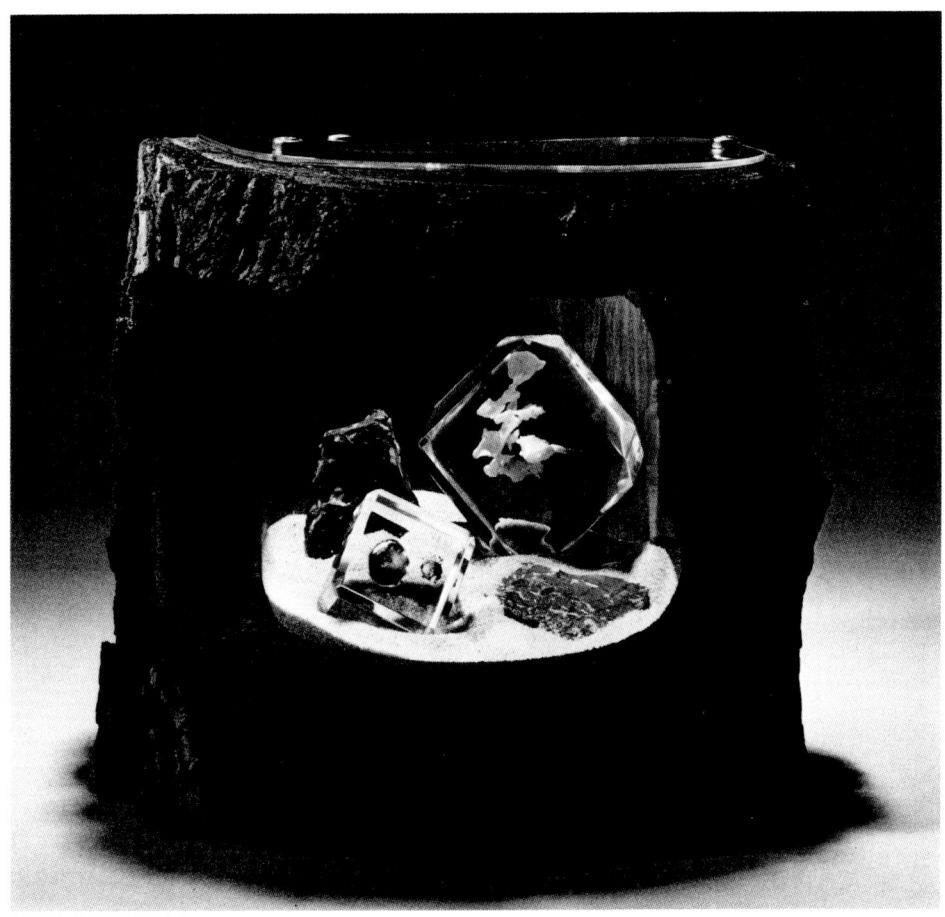

KATHY VARGAS

Valentine's Day/Day of the Dead #9, 1989–90
Hand-colored photograph
24 × 20 inches

"This series began as a remembrance of two friends who recently died of AIDS. One loved the Day of the Dead; the other met his mate on Valentine's Day. Their two favorite days seemed unfortunately 'appropriate' to AIDS…. At the time when each was dying, I sent *milagros* to their mates. [*Milagros* are tiny charms, in the form of metal hearts or body parts, which Vargas describes as "bribes offered to saints and deities, repayment for a miracle…and a prayer."] We all prayed for a miracle to save their lives, but it never came. After their deaths the prayers for them became transformed into prayers to them for others still awaiting miracles."

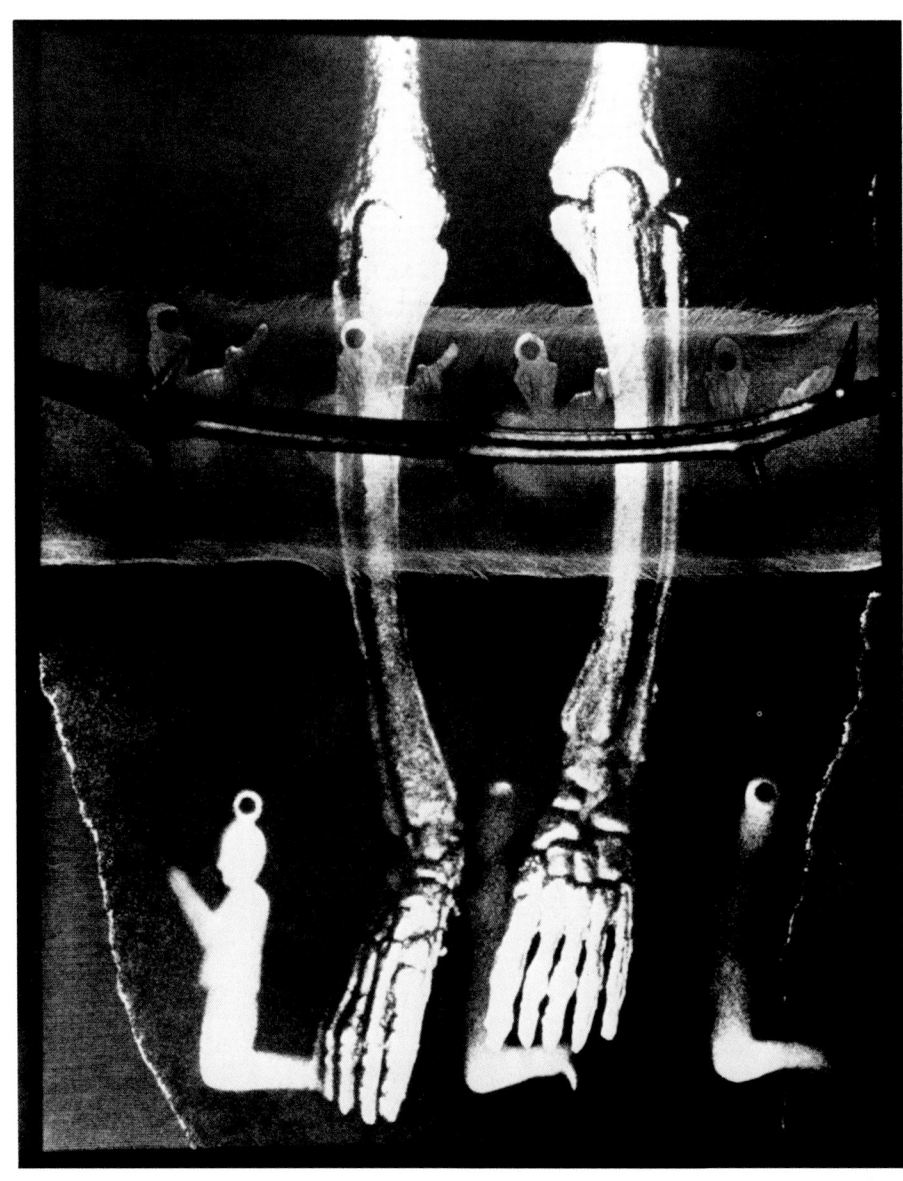

BRIAN WEIL

The Last Time Maria Saw Adriana, 1991
Gelatin silver print
42 × 42 inches

Photographer Brian Weil is an activist involved in ACT-UP/New York's needle-exchange program. His work documents the international scope of the AIDS epidemic and ranges from images of HIV-infected mothers in urban ghettoes in the United States to sex workers in Thailand. En masse, it is a graphic reminder of the extreme vulnerability of economically marginal populations to AIDS.

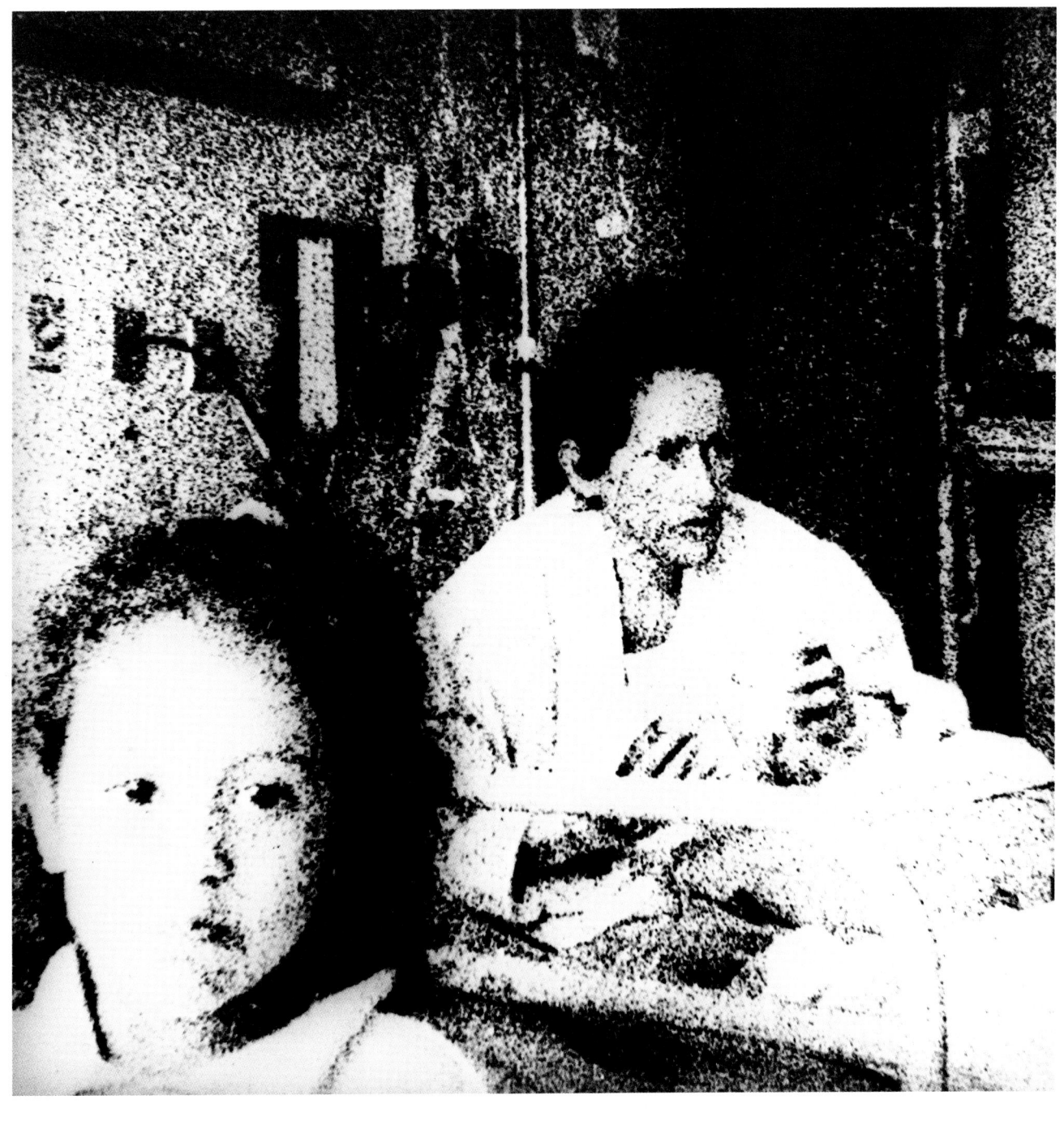

DAVID WOJNAROWICZ

Sex Series, 1988–89
1 of 8 gelatin silver prints
31 × 34¼ inches

The work of activist and PWA David Wojnarowicz has been at the center of several recent controversies about the public funding of sexually explicit, AIDS-related images. His angry catalogue essay attacking the role of the federal government and the Catholic Church in (mis)managing the AIDS crisis led John Frohnmayer—the then-new chairman of the National Endowment for the Arts—to withhold, and then reinstate, an NEA grant for *Witnesses: Against Our Vanishing*, an AIDS exhibition at Artists Space, in New York, in late 1989.

Fragmentary images from the *Sex Series*—culled from porno films—were pulled out of context by Donald Wildmon of the American Family Association and reprinted as an anti-NEA broadside. Wojnarowicz successfully sued Wildmon to end the illegal practice.

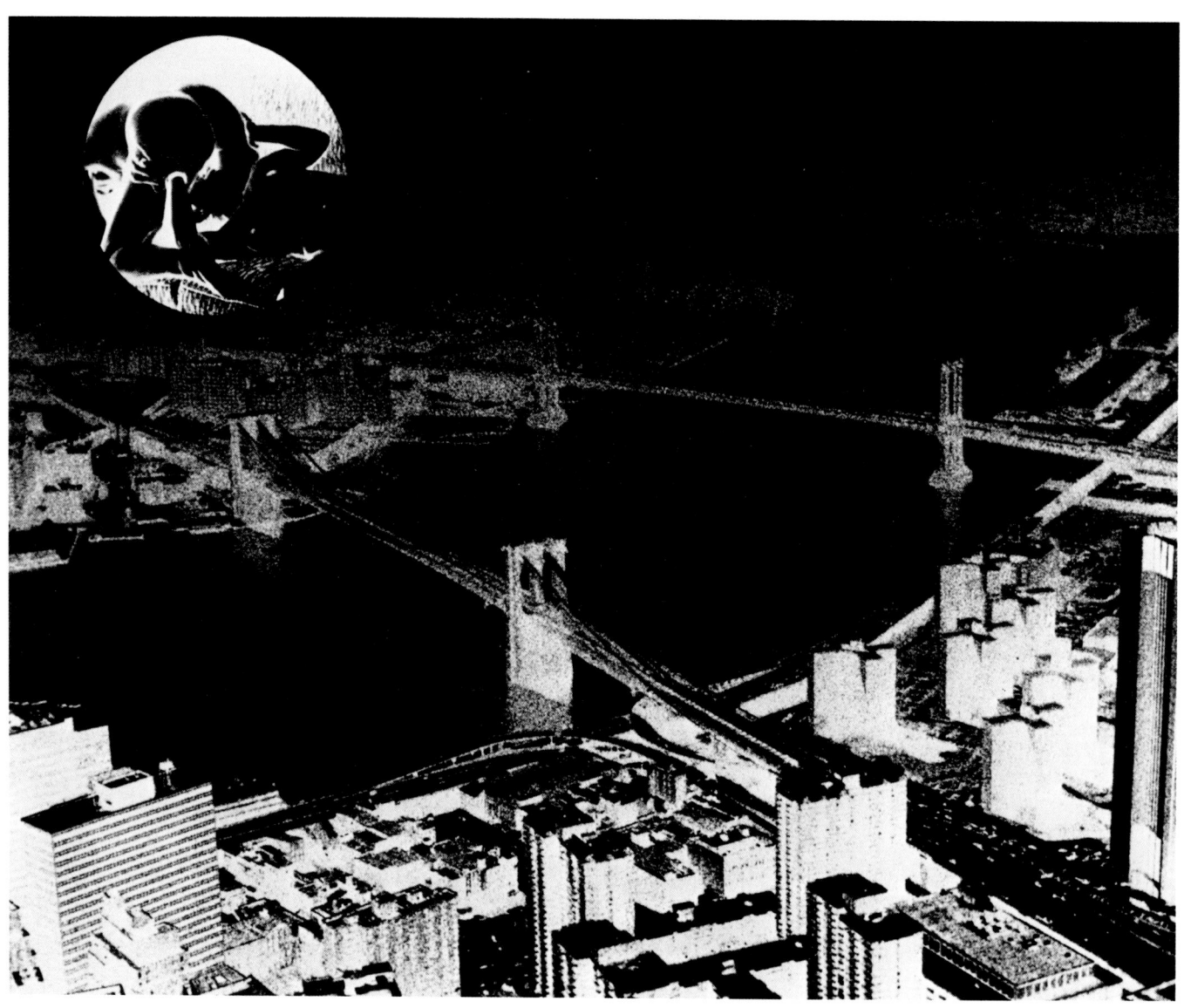

THOMAS WOODRUFF

*Chromatic Aberration,
Crying Clown-Brown*, 1990
Acrylic on canvas
42½ × 30 inches

Thomas Woodruff's series of self-portraits as a crying clown—his third body of AIDS-related paintings—invoke emotionally high-pitched, sometimes Victorian sources. His technical virtuosity transforms what might be mere sentiment into disturbing feeling.

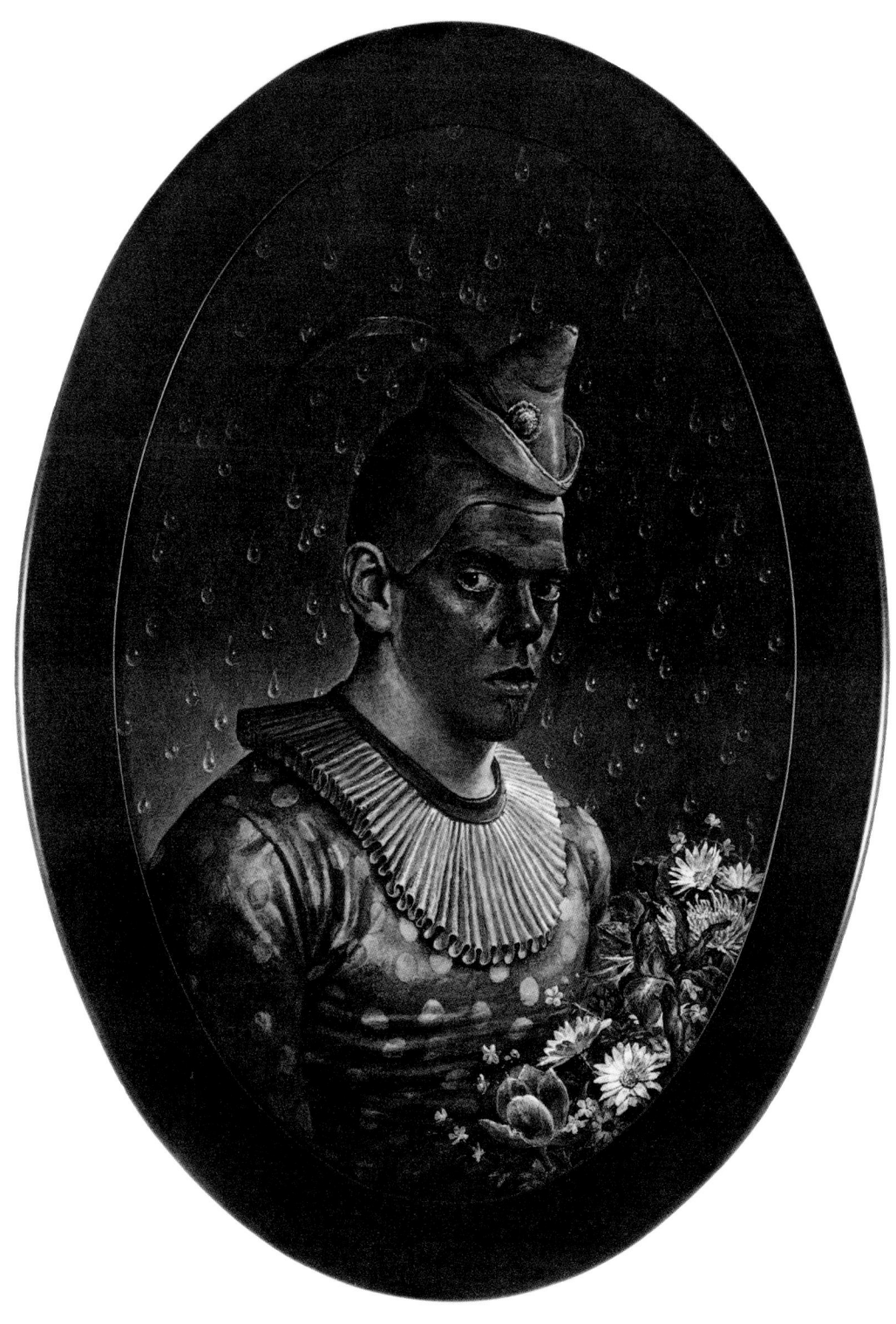

GRAN FURY

Still from *KISSING DOESN'T KILL: GREED AND INDIFFERENCE DO. CORPORATE GREED, GOVERNMENT INACTION AND PUBLIC INDIFFERENCE MAKE AIDS A POLITICAL CRISIS.*, 1991
VHS video compilation tape
120 seconds

Gran Fury is the art-making collective that emerged from ACT UP/New York. (ACT UP is the acronym for the AIDS Coalition to Unleash Power.) In November 1987, the as-yet-unnamed group created *Let the Record Show*, a potent and informative installation indicting the Reagan-Bush administration's inaction on AIDS, in the window of New York's New Museum of Contemporary Art. As ACT UP's propaganda office, Gran Fury produced numerous poster and sticker designs that effectively coupled the visual strategies of contemporary art and advertising.

Many of the collective's recent projects have been especially controversial. Commissioned as a publicly funded artwork for the sides of buses, a Benetton ad-inspired image of three kissing couples, *Kissing Doesn't Kill, Greed and Indifference Do*, generated heated controversy before finally being shown in Chicago in 1990. (A video version is included in this exhibition.) At the same time, Gran Fury's contribution to the Venice Bienale, the invitational international art exhibit, nearly led to Italian prosecution of the group for its criticism of the role of the Roman Catholic Church in the AIDS epidemic. Gran Fury now operates independently from ACT UP.

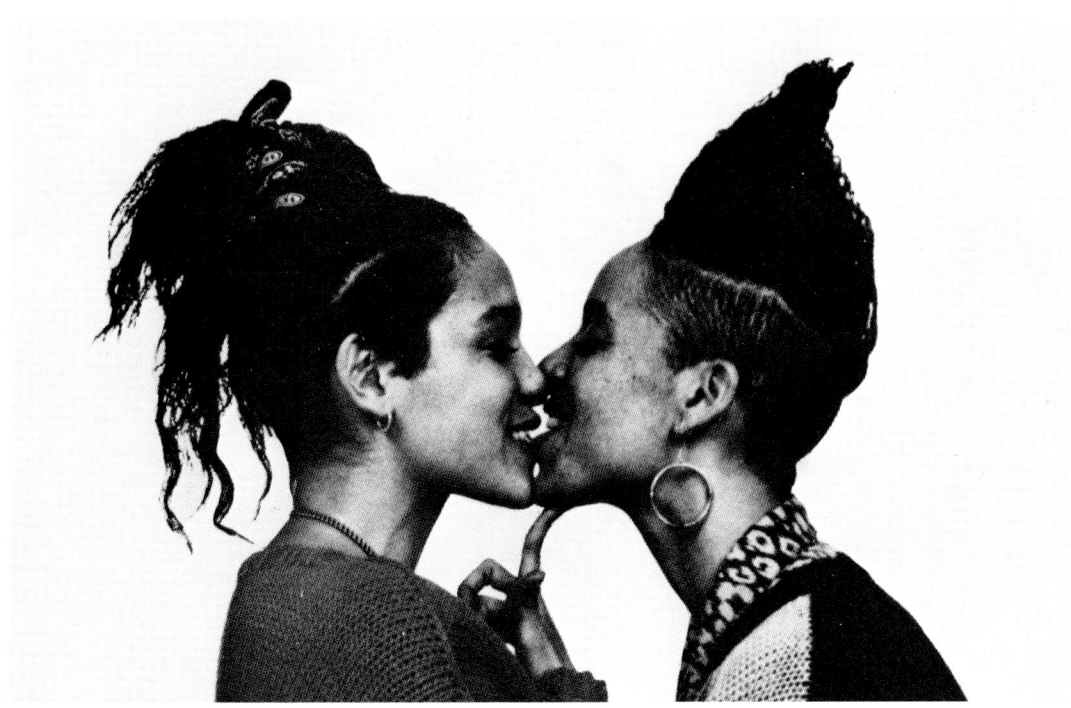

VIDEO DATA BANK

Video Against AIDS
Organized by Bill Horrigan and John Greyson
Produced by Video Data Bank
VHS video compilation tape
3 tapes, six hour collection

PROGRAM ONE, 114 MINUTES

PWA POWER

Survival of the Delirious
Michael Balser and Andy Fabo

Work Your Body
Gay Men's Health Crisis

DISCRIMINATION

The Second Epidemic
Amber Hollibaugh and Lisa Lebow

AIDS AND WOMEN

Safe Sex Slut
Carol Leigh

Cori: A Struggle for Life
Nina Sobell

Doctors, Liars and Women
Gay Men's Health Crisis

PROGRAM TWO, 119 MINUTES

RESISTANCE

ADS Epidemic
John Greyson

Snow Job
Barbara Hammer

We Are Not Republicans
Bob Huff

Stiff Sheets
John Goss

MOURNING

Mildred Pearson: When You Love a Person
Yannick Durand

Quilt
The NAMES Project

Danny
Stashu Kybartas

COMMUNITY EDUCATION

Se Met Ko
Patricia Benoit

PROGRAM THREE, 120 MINUTES

LOSS

A Plague Has Swept My City
Emjay Wilson

Gab
Ann Akiko Moriyasu

A
Andre Burke

This is Not an AIDS Advertisement
Isaac Julien

ANALYSIS

They are lost to vision altogether
Tom Kalin

Reframing AIDS
Pratibha Parmar

ACTIVISM

Another Man
Youth Against Monsterz

Testing the Limits NYC (Part 1)
Testing the Limits Collective

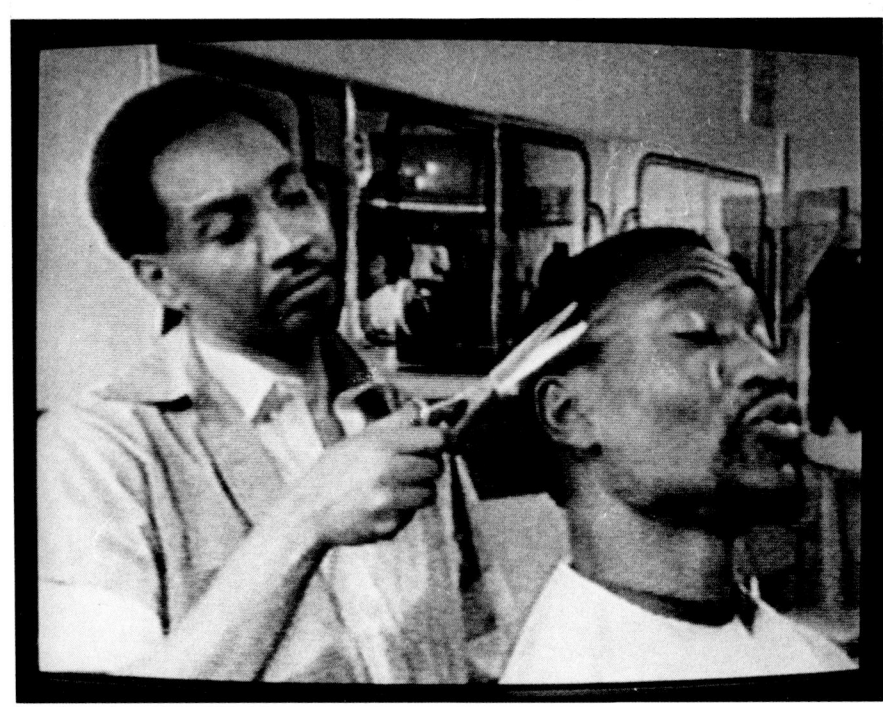

PATRICIA BENOIT *Se Met Ko*

VISUAL AIDS ARTISTS' CAUCUS

The Electric Blanket
2-carousel, 2-projector
slide program
Photo-documents by
David Armstrong
Sheyla Baykal
Donna Binder
Allen Clear
J.B. Diederich
Frank Fournier
Allen Frame
Tomas Gaspar
Nan Goldin
Steve Hart
Peter Hujar
Agosto Machado
Dona Ann McAdams
Tom McGovern
Scott Thode

Visual AIDS is an organization of art professionals whose purpose is to increase awareness and promote action about AIDS through educational projects and events. *The Electric Blanket* was produced for the second Day Without Art—a day of national action and mourning in response to the AIDS crisis held on December 1, 1990. The organizers put out an open call for AIDS-related photographic images. All submissions were projected during an evening-long program on a highly visible exterior wall of the Cooper Union in downtown Manhattan. The works presented here are a sampling of the works shown that night. For Day Without Art 1991, *The Electric Blanket* was exhibited throughout the United States. Members of the Artists' Caucus who organized *The Electric Blanket* were Allen Frame, Michael Goff, Nan Goldin, Paul H-O, and Joe Rudy.

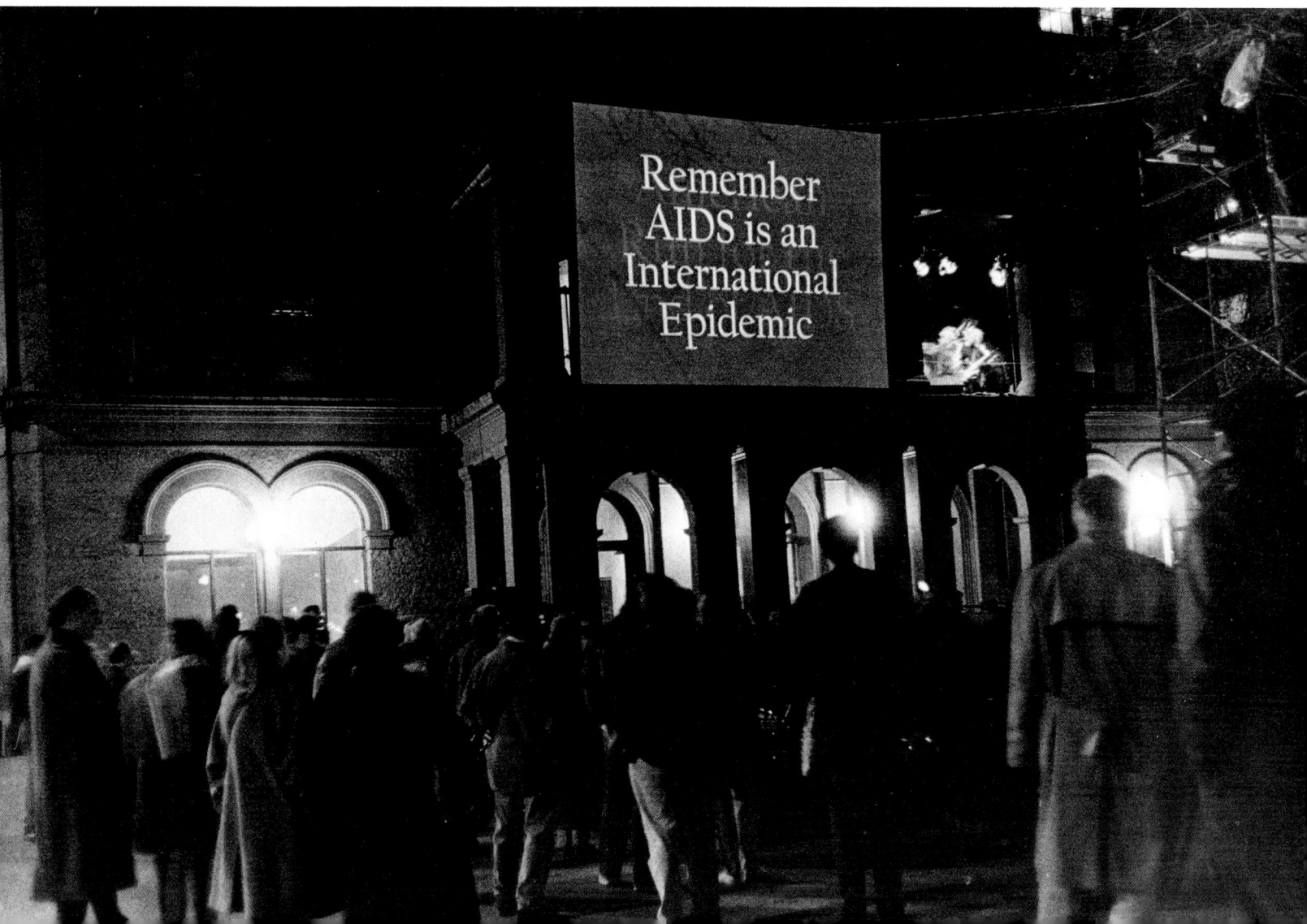

CHECKLIST

Height precedes
width precedes depth

(ART)ⁿ

In 1987, (Art)ⁿ consisted of Ellen Sandor, Stephan Meyers, Randy Johnson, Dan Sandin, and Jim Zanzi with special assistance from Dr. Roberta Glick. All artists reside in Chicago, IL. Date of first (Art)ⁿ collaboration: 1983

Messiah, 1987
PHSCologram sculpture
6 panels, 96 × 60 × 14 inches overall
Collection the artists and Feature, New York

ROSS BLECKNER

Born: 1949, New York, NY
Resides: New York, NY

Study for Internal Medicine, 1991
Oil on linen
4 panels, 18 × 14 inches each
36 × 28 inches overall
Collection the artist

KATHE BURKHART

Born: 1958, Martinsburg, WV
Resides: Brooklyn, NY

I Don't Have AIDS, 1990
From the series, *Liz Taylor (New York Post cover)*
Acrylic, modeling paste, and fake fur on canvas
78 × 78 inches
Collection the artist and Feature, New York

NANCY BURSON

Born: 1948, St. Louis, MO
Resides: New York, NY

Visualize This., 1991
Poster
18½ × 28½ inches
Courtesy Jayne H. Baum Gallery, New York

HIV-Infected T-Cell/Normal T-Cell, 1991
Diptych, silver dye-bleach (Cibachrome) prints
15 × 29 inches overall
Courtesy Jayne H. Baum Gallery, New York

STEVEN EVANS

Born: 1964, Key West, FL
Resides: New York, NY

Composition in Pink, Black, and White (variation), 1986
Gelatin silver prints and latex and oil paint on masonite and wood
60½ × 68 inches overall
Collection the artist

GENERAL IDEA

General Idea was formed in 1968.

A. A. Bronson
Born: 1946, Vancouver, Canada
Resides: Toronto, Canada and New York, NY

Felix Partz
Born: 1945, Winnipeg, Canada
Resides: Toronto, Canada

Jorge Zontal
Born: 1944, Parma, Italy
Resides: Toronto, Canada and New York, NY

Imagevirus (Times Square), 1989
Ektacolor RC print
30 × 20 inches
Courtesy the artists

Imagevirus (Posters), 1989
Ektacolor RC print
30 × 20 inches
Courtesy the artists

Imagevirus (Hamburg), 1989
Ektacolor RC print
30 × 20 inches
Courtesy the artists

Imagevirus (Amsterdam), 1991
Ektacolor RC print
30 × 20 inches
Courtesy the artists

Imagevirus (New York Subway), 1991
Ektacolor RC print
30 × 20 inches
Courtesy the artists

FELIX GONZALEZ-TORRES

Born: 1957, Guaimaro, Cuba
Resides: New York, NY

Untitled, 1988
Framed photostat
10½ × 11¾ inches
Courtesy the artist and Andrea Rosen Gallery, New York

GRAN FURY

Artists choose not to be identified
Date of first collaboration: 1988

KISSING DOESN'T KILL: GREED AND INDIFFERENCE DO. CORPORATE GREED, GOVERNMENT INACTION AND PUBLIC INDIFFERENCE MAKE AIDS A POLITICAL CRISIS., 1991

Produced by Gran Fury, New York
VHS video compilation tape
4 Public Service Announcements
30 seconds each, 120 seconds overall
Courtesy the artists

KEITH HARING

Born: 1958, Kutztown, PA
Died: 1990

Untitled (Billboard Design), 1989
Photostat
8 × 10 inches
Collection The Estate of Keith Haring

5 Things I Like about Safe Sex...(Part one) (Drawing for "High Risk"), 1989
Black felt-tip pen on paper
11 × 13 inches
Collection The Estate of Keith Haring

Silence=Death, 1989
Screenprint on paper
39 × 39 inches
Collection The Estate of Keith Haring

ADRIAN KELLARD

Born: 1959, New Rochelle, NY
Died: 1991

The Promise/I Will Never Leave You, 1989
Carved wood with paint
75 × 45 × 2 inches
Courtesy the Estate of Adrian Kellard

PETER KUNZ-OPFERSEI

Born: 1944, Opfersei Hergiswil, Switzerland
Died: 1988

Book of Drawings #1, 1987-88
Black ink on paper, 85 drawings
7 × 5 inches each page
Collection Raymond Jacobs

Book of Drawings #2, 1987-88
Mixed media on paper, 39 pieces
9⅛ × 6⅜ inches each page
Collection Raymond Jacobs

Book of Drawings #3, 1987-88
Black ink on paper, 120 drawings
6 × 4 inches each page
Collection Raymond Jacobs

Book of Drawings #4, 1987-88
Mixed media on paper, 80 drawings
9¼ × 6⅛ inches each page
Collection Raymond Jacobs

RUDY LEMCKE

Born: 1951, St. Louis, MO
Resides: San Francisco, CA

Garden, 1988
Architectural model for AIDS monument
(subway station overview)
¼ scale model, 21 × 30 × 9 inches
Collection the artist

Garden, 1988
Architectural model for AIDS monument
½ scale model, 24 × 24 × 7 inches
Collection the artist

ROBERT MAPPLETHORPE

Born: 1946, Floral Park, NY
Died: 1989

Self-Portrait, 1988
Gelatin silver print
24 × 20 inches
Collection The Robert Mapplethorpe Foundation
Courtesy Robert Miller Gallery, New York

PAUL MARCUS

Born: 1953, Bronx, NY
Resides: New York, NY

Maze of AIDS, 1989
Oil on wood and audio cassette
Painting: 72 × 96 inches
Recording: 3:55 minutes
Courtesy P.P.O.W., New York

DUANE MICHALS

Born: 1932, McKeesport, PA
Resides: New York, NY

The Dream of Flowers, 1986
4 gelatin silver prints
5 × 7 inches each
Courtesy Sidney Janis Gallery, New York

DONALD MOFFETT

Born: 1955, San Antonio, TX
Resides: New York, NY

Call the White House, 1990
Back-lit Ciba-transparency
40 × 60 × 7 inches
Courtesy the artist

FRANK MOORE

Born: 1953, New York, NY
Resides: New York, NY

Bubble Bath, 1990
Oil on canvas with mixed media
83½ × 99½ inches
Collection the artist

ELLEN B. NEIPRIS

Born: 1961, Boston, MA
Resides: Brooklyn, NY

AIDS Vigil (New York City), 1985
Gelatin silver print
11 × 14 inches
Collection the artist

Lesbian and Gay March (Washington, D.C.), 1987
Gelatin silver print
11 × 14 inches
Collection the artist

ACT UP, Republican National Convention (New Orleans), 1988
Gelatin silver print
11 × 14 inches
Collection the artist

Lesbian and Gay Anti-Violence Demonstration (New York City), 1991
Gelatin silver print
11 × 14 inches
Collection the artist

DIANE NEUMAIER

Born: 1946, Minneapolis, MN
Resides: New York, NY

Untitled, 1988
From the series, *Street Graphic Interventions*
Black-and-white resin-coated print
16 × 20 inches
Collection the artist

Untitled, 1988
From the series, *Street Graphic Interventions*
Black-and-white resin-coated print
16 × 20 inches
Collection the artist

NICHOLAS AND BEBE NIXON

Nicholas Nixon
Born: 1947, Detroit, MI
Resides: Cambridge, MA

Bebe Nixon
Born: 1949, Providence, RI
Resides: Cambridge, MA

Laverne Colebut, 1988-89
8 gelatin silver prints and 1 text panel
Prints: 8 × 10 inches each
Courtesy Zabriskie Gallery, New York

GYPSY RAY

Born: 1949, Kewanee, IL
Resides: Santa Cruz, CA

Zenobia and Jon, 1986
Gelatin silver print and text
20 × 16 inches
Collection the artist

Wesley Harris, 1987
Gelatin silver print and text
20 × 16 inches
Collection the artist

ROD RHODES

Born: 1944, Marshalltown, IA
Died: 1989

Stations of the Cross X, Stripping of Christ, 1988
Wood, glass, and felt
26 × 26 × 6¾ inches
Collection Andreas Weber

JANE ROSETT

Born: 1961, New York, NY
Resides: Brooklyn, NY

Untitled, 1990
From the series, *Belle Glade, Florida*
Ektacolor RC print
16 × 20 inches
Collection the artist

Untitled, 1990
From the series, *Belle Glade, Florida*
Ektacolor RC print
16 × 20 inches
Collection the artist

Untitled, 1990
From the series, *Belle Glade, Florida*
Ektacolor RC print
16 × 20 inches
Collection the artist

Untitled, 1990
From the series, *Belle Glade, Florida*
Ektacolor RC print
16 × 20 inches
Collection the artist

JOHN SAPP

Born: 1947, Houston, TX
Resides: New York, NY

Adam and I Finally Went to Key West, 1989
Charcoal on paper
60 × 84 inches
Collection the artist

DUI SEID

Born: 1945, Greenville, MS
Resides: New York, NY

Scum, 1989
Plastic, medical supplies, and text
96 × 72 × 6 inches
Collection the artist

JO SHANE

Born: 1955, Boston, MA
Resides: New York, NY

President's Choice (This is a P.C. Product), 1991
Mixed-media installation
63¾ × 78 × 78 inches overall
Collection the artist

ROSALIND SOLOMON

Born: 1930, Highland Park, IL
Resides: New York, NY

Garden, New York, 1988
From the series, *Portraits in the Time of AIDS*
Gelatin silver print
32 × 32 inches
Collection the artist

Lenny with his Parents, Brooklyn, New York, 1987
From the series, *Portraits in the Time of AIDS*
Gelatin silver print
32 × 32 inches
Collection the artist

MASAMI TERAOKA

Born: 1936, Onomichi, Japan
Resides: Waimanalo, HI

AIDS Series/Geisha and AIDS Nightmare, 1989-90
Watercolor on canvas
106¼ × 74 inches
Courtesy Pamela Auchincloss Gallery, New York

MAX (TORQUE) = DOUG [(BRUNO) HAMMETT]

Born: 1963, Los Angeles, CA
Resides: Pasadena, CA

Re-Circulate, 1990
From the series, *Sleeping Beauty*
Mixed-media sculpture
Sculpture: 11 × 10 × 11 inches
Collection the artist

KATHY VARGAS

Born: 1950, San Antonio, TX
Resides: San Antonio, TX

Valentine's Day/Day of the Dead #9, 1989-90
Hand-colored photograph
24 × 20 inches
Collection the artist

Valentine's Day/Day of the Dead #14, 1989-1990
Hand-colored photograph
23½ × 13½ inches
Collection the artist

VIDEO DATA BANK

Video Against AIDS
Organized by Bill Horrigan and John Greyson
Produced by the Video Data Bank, Chicago
VHS video compilation tapes
3-tape, 6-hour collection
Courtesy Video Data Bank, Chicago

VISUAL AIDS ARTISTS CAUCUS

The Electric Blanket
2-carousel, 2-projector slide program
Photo-documents by David Armstrong, Sheyla Baykal, Donna Binder, Allen Clear, J.B. Diederich, Frank Fournier, Allen Frame, Tomas Gaspar, Nan Goldin, Steve Hart, Peter Hujar, Agosto Machado, Dona Ann McAdams, Tom McGovern, and Scott Thode
Courtesy Visual AIDS Artists' Caucus, New York

BRIAN WEIL

Born: 1954, Chicago, IL
Resides: New York, NY

Male Sex Workers, Bangkok, Thailand, 1990
Gelatin silver print
42 × 42 inches
Collection the artist

The Last Time Maria Saw Adriana, 1991
Gelatin silver print
42 × 42 inches
Collection the artist

DAVID WOJNAROWICZ

Born: 1954, Red Bank, NJ
Resides: New York, NY

Sex Series, 1988-89
8 gelatin silver prints
31 × 34¼ inches each
Courtesy P.P.O.W., New York

THOMAS WOODRUFF

Born: 1957, New Rochelle, NY
Resides: New York, NY

Chromatic Aberration, Crying Clown-Brown, 1990
Acrylic on canvas
42½ × 30 inches
Courtesy P.P.O.W., New York

REPRODUCTION CREDITS
John Cooper III 56
Courtesy Feature, New York 33
Courtesy Jayne H. Baum Gallery, New York 34
Courtesy Pamela Auchincloss Gallery, New York 58
Courtesy Sidney Janis Gallery, New York 44-45
Courtesy The Estate of Keith Haring 38
D. James Dee 46
A. Gridley Graves 32, 36-37, 39, 47, 50, 52-53
Doug Hammett 59
Dona Ann McAdams 67
Adam Reich 43, 62-63

In addition to all other copyrights and reservations pertaining to works published in this catalogue and held by living artists, their estates, publications, and/or foundations, and in addition to the photographers and the sources of photographic material other than those indicated in the captions the following are mentioned: Robert Mapplethorpe: © 1988 by The Estate of Robert Mapplethorpe. Ellen B. Neipris: © by Ellen B. Neipris. Diane Neumaier: © by Diane Neumaier. Gypsy Ray: © by Gypsy Ray. Rosalind Solomon: © by Rosalind Solomon. Kathy Vargas: © by Kathy Vargas. Brian Weil: © by Brian Weil.

© 1991 Independent Curators Incorporated
799 Broadway, Suite 205
New York, NY 10003

All rights reserved. No part of this catalogue may be reproduced without written permission except in the case of brief quotations in critical articles or reviews.

Editorial Consultant: Marybeth Sollins
Design and Typography: Russell Hassell
Lithography: The Studley Press
Limited edition of 1,500

Library of Congress
Catalogue Card Number: 91-76797
ISBN: 0-916365-34-3